OVERCOMING ANGER IN YOUR RELATIONSHIP

OVERCOMING
ANGER
IN YOUR
RELATIONSHIP

HOW TO BREAK THE CYCLE
OF ARGUMENTS, PUT-DOWNS,
AND STONY SILENCES

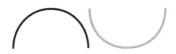

W. ROBERT NAY, PhD

THE GUILFORD PRESS
New York   London

© 2010 The Guilford Press
A Division of Guilford Publications, Inc.
72 Spring Street, New York, NY 10012
www.guilford.com

Printed in the United States of America

This book is printed on acid-free paper.

Last digit is print number: 9   8   7   6   5   4   3   2   1

Library of Congress Cataloging-in-Publication Data

Nay, W. Robert.
    Overcoming anger in your relationship : how to break the cycle of
arguments, put-downs, and stony silences / W. Robert Nay.
        p.   cm.
    Includes bibliographical references and index.
    ISBN 978-1-60623-283-5 (pbk. : alk. paper)
    ISBN 978-1-60623-642-0 (hardcover : alk. paper)
    1. Anger. 2. Interpersonal conflict. 3. Interpersonal relations.
4. Couples—Psychology.   I. Title.
    BF575.A5N384 2010
    152.4′7—dc22

                                                    2010001686

To my major professor, mentor, and friend,
Henry Earl Adams, PhD

All who knew him and became his students
miss him terribly

Lives of great men all remind us
We can make our lives sublime,
And, departing, leave behind us
Footprints in the sands of time.
—HENRY WADSWORTH LONGFELLOW

CONTENTS

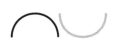

PART I

Five Steps to Change in Your Relationship

ACKNOWLEDGMENTS

First, I want to thank Kitty Moore, Executive Editor at The Guilford Press. Following the success of *Taking Charge of Anger: How to Resolve Conflict, Sustain Relationships, and Express Yourself without Losing Control*, which I wrote for those who need help in understanding and managing anger in their lives and relationships, she suggested that I write a book addressing the needs of the partners of those angry individuals. The goal was to provide ideas for identifying the negative impact of anger and to craft, express, and sustain firm boundaries with the angry partner as to what was acceptable behavior in the future. Setting such boundaries early on would halt the slippery slope of many relationships into serious communication breakdown or verbal and even physical abuse. A worthy goal and an important project to strengthen, if not salvage, troubled relationships. Thanks for the vision and the continuing support.

Next I want to thank my editor, Chris Benton, with whom I worked closely during each phase of this project. This is the second book on which I have had the privilege of working with Chris, who is a wonderful wordsmith, an attentive and sustaining coach, an insightful "therapist" at those junctures when you really need emotional support and some outright praise, and a great writer.

I also want to thank the hundreds of individuals and couples who have permitted me to enter into their lives at a difficult time. I have learned so much from working with you. Also, I am thankful for the many professional counselors and therapists who have attended my workshops on anger over the past decade. I have learned much from the give-and-take of your questions and comments.

Finally, I would not have had the stamina to get through some serious health problems and continue onward to the end of this project were it not for my dear wife, Joyce, an outstanding therapist in her own right and a great life partner.

INTRODUCTION

Amy loves her husband but doesn't love being around him these days. The couple can't seem to spend an hour together without Ed's getting tense and irritable because one thing or another has gone wrong.

Ryan knows Kate is "hot-tempered," but he's sick of being called "a loser" and other names just because Kate is supposedly under so much stress.

Sandy always found the verbal sparring in her relationship kind of exciting—until Ty started grabbing her arm in a way that makes her wonder: Could Ty ever hurt her?

Charles never dreamed he'd be tempted to have an affair. Now that he's fantasizing about it, he's torn between guilt and his own anger at Sonya for regularly holing herself up in their bedroom to make him pay for some transgression she refuses to name.

Anger can gain a foothold in the most loving relationship. One day you wake up and wonder what happened to the happy union you once had. Where did the pleasure you once took in each other's company go? What happened to the trust and closeness? And what is your partner so mad about anyway?

If you love someone whose anger has started to erode the intimacy

1

between you, and you wonder how much more you—and the relationship—can take, this book offers hope. Anger can shake the very foundation of your relationship and pose a serious threat to your personal well-being. Of course you want it to stop. In fact you've undoubtedly tried to make your partner's anger stop, to no avail. Fortunately, being unable to force your partner to change is not a dead end. There's a lot that *you* can change, even without cooperation from your angry partner, that will protect you from becoming anger's victim and restore your own well-being. This book will show you how.

Most people I counsel want to preserve their relationship too. This person who seems consumed by ire or rage is the one they've come to trust and value more than anyone else. The partnership has already produced cherished memories, shared joys and tragedies, possibly children, and a love that was probably thriving until anger came along. Even if your relationship seems in danger of disintegrating, it's probably not too late to put it back together. The prognosis for the partnership depends in part on your partner, but with a strong lead from you, there's a good chance your partner will follow and repairs can be made.

Of course, if you are the victim of physical violence or other abuse, the situation is entirely different. I urge you to put your own safety and welfare (and that of any children) first, and only after doing so consider whether the relationship can be salvaged. Fortunately, most people I meet who no longer know how to live with an angry partner just want the peace and comfort of their former life with the person they love so much. Most people who are struggling with a partner's chronic anger are not battered, but they are certainly demoralized and depleted by:

- Trying to reason with someone who agrees to change, apologizes, and then goes back to the same unacceptable behavior.

- Arranging their whole life to avoid triggering their partner's anger.

- Taking responsibility for making their partner mad.

- Trying to forgive and explain away their partner's anger.

Sound familiar? When it's the person you love most who imposes his or her anger on you, it's easy to get roped into trying to compensate, ride it out, extend empathy, and help your partner destress. The trouble is that by doing so over and over you may signal your partner that hostility, yelling, name-calling, sarcasm, and other inappropriate ways of expressing anger are perfectly fine with you: your partner can feel free to keep indulging in this misbehavior. When that happens, the pattern becomes entrenched. No amount of cajoling or pleading, threatening or demanding will force your partner to change. You're left to wonder how things got so bad and how in the world you're going to get out of this mess.

If this sounds like you, you can benefit from a straightforward approach I've developed that will help you extricate yourself from the grip of *reaction* mode and start taking *action* to reject behavior that you don't find acceptable. It all comes down to taking a close look at yourself:

- How your partner's anger is affecting you and how you react to it.

- How you want to be treated differently.

- What thinking habits you have that keep you stuck in accepting the unacceptable.

- How you can express what you expect to protect your new boundaries and deny your partner any reward for anger.

Thirty years ago I became interested in understanding the emotion of anger in relationships: what triggers it, how it seems to develop into many different "faces" of expression, and how to manage it so it doesn't manage you (me). I have worked with hundreds of couples when anger has become a roadblock to intimacy. I have trained more than three thousand mental health professionals in the principles and procedures of managing anger and learned from their feedback and ideas. I developed a six-step strategy for managing anger based on this work and the latest research into anger and conflict in relationships. While my book *Taking Charge of Anger* (see Suggested Resources) addressed the needs of a person whose anger is getting out of control, it did not offer guidance to Amy, Ryan, Sandy, Charles, or you—the partners who are living day to day with unacceptable expressions of anger.

That's why I wrote this book. In the following pages you'll learn that when *you* make changes, your partner can no longer use his or her old anger tactics to dump anger on you. You are no longer reacting in the same way, so your partner is faced with a dilemma: keep doing the same old thing *without* getting the same old reaction from you, or change. You cannot control your partner's decision, but you will immediately feel better about your own life when you no longer react in the old ways. You are changing and inviting your partner to join you in a new, more peaceful, and intimate relationship.

I'm confident that you'll find the effort worth making. Anger is a slippery slope. What starts out as "innocent" teasing, "joking" sarcasm, occasional flares of temper, or scattershot irritation can mushroom into anger that's more intense, more frequent, and more intentionally hurtful. A major goal of this book is to illustrate how choosing to make no changes yourself can inadvertently allow your partner to progress from being chronically crabby to verbally abusive and then even physically violent. This may seem like an alarmist position, but those of us who counsel people entangled in anger have seen it happen again and again: inappropriate anger begets even more inappropriate anger. And if you're in the firing line, that means your well-being is increasingly at risk.

Make no mistake about it: inappropriate expressions of anger are destructive—to you and to your relationship. What you may wish you could explain away as unintentional and stress-related can actually be psychological abuse, which research shows is harmful to your self-esteem on its own. And over time, the research also shows, it can transform into physical abuse.

So if you're beginning to feel you can't live with your partner's anger anymore, now is the time to get out of the firing line and back to the life you deserve. I hope the strategies and advice that follow will help.

PART I

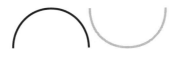

Five Steps
to Change
in Your
Relationship

1

UNDERSTANDING AND CONFRONTING ANGER

The Promise of Change

Sarah hated it when Jeff was "stressed out" as he called it. He got loudly critical—of her, the kids, the driver ahead of him, her parents, and anyone else who annoyed him. He was impatient and irritable, and when he wasn't on the attack he became very distant. Anything that went "wrong" or got "out of control" in his eyes seemed to set him off, and Sarah never knew when that might happen or what to expect of her husband. "It sometimes feels like I turn my own life inside out to make sure he won't get upset," she told her closest friends. When her friends had heard that lament dozens of times and asked her what she intended to do about it, she sighed and said, "I guess I'll just live with it."

Frank admitted he had a bad temper. He conceded that when he lost it he was prone to cursing and yelling and that he had called his fiancée, Linda, "stupid," "limited," "a moron," and other names. But he wasn't the one with the anger problem, he insisted. It was Linda who caused the whole problem by constantly comparing him to his father, an alcoholic who regularly beat his mother. Getting angry back at her was the only way he could get her to stop criticizing him, he said. But as time went on, cursing and yelling had given way to pushing and shoving and physically restraining Linda to keep her from leaving the room or the house.

John and Nancy had been chipping away at their marriage with a kind of cold, quiet violence for several years. It wasn't unusual for John to get an icy greeting from his wife after they both got home from work. Or her mood would suddenly shift after he thought they'd been having a nice evening together, and she'd slip off to the bedroom without explanation and without answering him when he tried to call after her. No matter how much he pleaded, she wouldn't tell him what was wrong or what he'd done: "I just want to be alone," she'd insist. "Nothing's wrong, but I don't want to talk—just let me be." Eventually he would—and then he'd decide to make Nancy "pay" by doing a little withdrawing of his own, leaving the house for parts unknown for hours at a time. Lately he'd started skipping the pleading part of the game and just left.

HOW IS ANGER DAMAGING YOUR LIFE?

Are any of these couples familiar? If you're living with or close to someone who is often irritable or blows up regularly but unpredictably, who demeans you with sarcasm or put-downs, who is verbally aggressive or threatening, or who withdraws and withholds attention to express anger, you know how damaging it can be. Sarah started having tension headaches so frequently that her physician prescribed a muscle relaxer and an antidepressant to "calm" her nerves. John alternated between deep hurt and outrage: Why was Nancy treating him like a stranger, as if it wasn't worth explaining his transgressions to him because they were never going to see each other again? Linda was becoming afraid of the man she loved. How much worse would Frank's temper get once they were married?

Whether a loved one's anger is direct—like Jeff's and Frank's—or indirect, like Nancy's, being on the receiving end of anger is tremendously hurtful. It leaves scars that don't heal easily, often because the angry person typically denies that his or her anger is a problem or fails to take any responsibility for these episodes. Do any of these excuses for anger sound familiar?

"If you would just stop nagging me, I wouldn't get so upset."

"I'm not the one with the problem—it's your insecurity that's the problem."

"You're just overreacting again. Get over it!"

Excuses like these are insidious. You are not perfect either, but you *know* in your heart that your partner's anger is out of proportion to whatever situation seems to have triggered it. You *know* that your partner needs to take responsibility for the way he or she expresses high emotion like anger. Yet after an outburst or a siege, many people start to wonder whether it's true that they're to blame. When all you want is to avoid a repeat of your partner's anger, the idea that a little less nagging or a little more self-confidence on your part might make all the difference can start to seem pretty reasonable. Watching yourself for signs that you're over-reacting might not seem like such a big deal. If making changes on your own will do the trick, maybe that's not such a bad idea.

If you've rationalized like this, you're on the right track but going in the wrong direction.

Changes you make *can* set the stage for your relationship with an angry partner to change, *but not changes designed to accommodate the way your partner is expressing anger.* You're probably reading this book because you've made lots of attempts to change the way your partner acts, and they haven't worked. Maybe you've started to arrange your lives together to avoid things that seem to trigger your partner's anger. Sarah's list of things she would do to "keep Jeff calm" seemed to grow every week. She'd try to keep the children quiet and send them to bed as early as possible so he wouldn't get angry at their "noise" and demands. She avoided going to her parents' home with him as much as possible because they "annoyed" him and she did not want her mother and father to feel her husband's distaste for them. People often try such accommodations after their more direct attempts to change their partner's behavior have failed. Sadly, such measures often send the implicit message that the angry person's way of expressing anger is appropriate. *It is not.* And the only thing that does set the stage for the relationship to change, as you'll see in this book, is to make that clear by changing the way you *react.*

Most of my clients get trapped in a vicious cycle of anger because they keep trying the same old tactics. They get angry back. They retaliate in some other way, like John's showing Nancy that "two can play that game" by withdrawing from her whenever she withdraws from him. They try reasoning with their partner. When nothing works, they may decide they really must be to blame. After all, it's not as if their partner is a terrible person, angry all the time. "He's a great husband when he's calm, and I love him," Sarah would say when her friends asked why she didn't just leave Jeff. Linda wanted to marry Frank; she knew they loved each other and that, ironically, their attachment and passion were evident in how reactive and emotional they got in their endless arguments. Somehow, then, these partners found a way to "live" with their loved one's anger. But because their reactions to their partners stayed the same, the outcomes stayed the same. Anger continued to rule their lives.

Eventually, a partner's anger becomes a burden too heavy to bear. You may very well feel now that it's unfair to have to adjust your own life to your partner's anger, that it's becoming too costly for you. Have you ever changed your plans to accommodate your partner because you were apprehensive that she "couldn't stand" or "couldn't cope" with a situation without getting upset and angry? Has the threat of your husband's anger prevented you from inviting a certain relative or friend over for fear that he might say or do something in anger that would embarrass you? Do you sometimes avoid discussing certain topics that you know are triggers for his anger, even though you very much want him to know how you feel? These and many other possible adjustments can greatly affect the quality of your life. You may find yourself resenting this person for the limits his or her anger seems to place on your choices, outcomes, and possibilities.

You'll have an opportunity to assess how you react emotionally and how you currently cope with this person's anger in Chapter 2, but it's probably already clear to you that you're paying a big price that has started to feel unacceptable. Like the sand gradually wearing away the painted finish on the bottom of a boat, living with an angry person begins to wear away at one's most personal self. Perhaps you've noticed that you feel more depressed than you used to feel and sometimes have sad thoughts of leaving this person. Or your self-esteem may have taken a hit as you suffer through repeated episodes of hostility or aggression that you don't deserve but can't seem to alter. Maybe you feel like your life has changed drastically and you have no idea how you got where you are today.

THE MANY FACES OF ANGER

Anger makes inroads into intimate relationships in part because it comes in many shapes and sizes that we don't always identify as anger. There's the yelling, intense version that most of us think of when we say someone is angry—the kind of anger that is depleting Sarah's reservoir of commitment to her marriage and that may keep Frank and Linda from getting married at all. As is usually the case with Jeff, this expression can take the form of plain hostility about why things are so slow or frustration when a line is too long. Or it can manifest itself in its more sinister form of outright nastiness and aggression, as with Frank. In any form, loud and intense anger is no fun for the beholder (you) and most often isn't a picnic for the angry person. Most of us don't like to be around others who are outwardly and intensely angry, and some of us react in ways that are incredibly unhelpful and even damaging to ourselves. Linda is amazed to find herself right in there, battling it out with Frank "like some sort of thug." She doesn't like the person she sees in the mirror these days.

Then there is anger that doesn't look like anger at all. Let's imagine I'm angry because you didn't show up for a lunch date on time. Instead of calmly telling you how I feel (confused and irritated), I make out like nothing is wrong. When you try to talk to me, I'm quiet and respond minimally, making you do all the work. Pretty soon you ask, "What's the matter?" I reply, "What do you mean? Why *nothing's* wrong!" This is a way of being passively angry. While not loud and obnoxious, passive–aggression is toxic in its own special way. You know I'm mad, but I won't admit it and withhold what you want.

Anger is not inappropriate in and of itself. But there are inappropriate ways to express it that fall into certain general categories defined in the box on the next page. Whether anger is expressed in active, intense, and forceful ways or is shown in passive and indirect comments and actions, each of these anger styles is a roadblock to good communication and intimacy in your relationship. Your partner may express anger in just one of these ways or in several ways. Some people use one face of anger at home and another in public or at work. Or they seem perfectly capable of expressing anger appropriately with others but not with us. It's important to understand which face of anger your partner is wearing at any given time so that you know how to alter your reaction to it in a way that protects you from further damage and, as I said earlier, sets the stage for change in your relationship. The stories told in this book will help you identify your partner's particular faces of anger and look specifically at how to deal with each one you may be encountering. Even more important, though, is understanding how anger can affect the behavior of both partners.

Faces of Anger

Face of anger	Characteristics to look for
Passive–aggression	Withholds praise, attention, or affection. May "forget" or fail to follow through on commitments. Withholds intimacy when upset. Engages in actions known to upset the other person. Chronic lateness.
Sarcasm	Makes "humorous" or cutting remarks about others. Reveals embarrassing personal information to others or causes public humiliation. Uses a tone of voice and manner that convey disgust or disapproval.
Cold anger	Withdraws from the other person for periods of time. Avoids intimacy. Refuses to reveal what is wrong. Tends to avoid emotional discussion when angry.
Hostility	Conveys an inner intensity, raised voice—seems more stressed out. Acts time-impatient. Shows visible signs of frustration and annoyance with others who don't move fast enough or who fail to meet high expectations for competence or performance.
Aggression	Raises voice, verbally loud and/or abusive. Curses, uses name-calling, and blames. Has thoughts or mental pictures of hurting another. Acts out anger with touching, pushing, blocking, or hitting.

UNDERSTANDING THE IMPACT OF ANGER ON YOUR RELATIONSHIP

Are you, like Sarah, living with a partner's anger that has become a constant source of discomfort for you? Do you feel like your entire life is now crafted to avoid, prevent, or control your partner's anger? Or do you feel like your partner's anger is a maelstrom that pulls you in, making you join in the anger and leading to an endless series of arguments, battles of will, and scorekeeping? Sarah is marching to Jeff's angry tune. She's trying to find a way to live with the circumstances she hasn't been able to change, but she's so stressed out by the tension that she can't think straight. The other couples are all following each other's lead and can't seem to change their routines. The unhelpful expression of one partner sets the stage for the other. Following Frank's lead, Frank and Linda are both getting more and more physically aggressive. Nancy and John both withdraw. All of these people have gotten lost in these inappropriate expressions of anger; no one is able to convey what really needs to be said or to resolve conflicts that simmer under the surface.

For John and Nancy the problem wasn't so much *what* ideas, feelings, and needs their anger was preventing them from conveying but *how* their communications fell apart. When Nancy got angry at John, her anger upset her further. She'd been raised to believe it wasn't right to feel, much less express, strong anger, and so she clammed up, justifying her cold silence by telling herself her husband should know her well enough to know why she was angry anyway—she shouldn't have to explain. John felt so hurt and rejected that his pride was injured along with his feelings, and *he* decided he shouldn't have to explain, so he withdrew more himself.

It's only natural to get angry in response to what you believe is unfair anger aimed at you. It's only reasonable that, when it feels like the rug is pulled out from under you by your partner's anger, your partner take responsibility for changing the drill. Right?

How We Get Entangled

If you are in a well-established and loving relationship with this person, it makes sense that you would want him or her to be motivated to make some changes. How have you tried to provide that motivation when your partner doesn't seem to have it?

Taking the direct approach—letting your partner know clearly that you're unhappy with this angry "face" and that he or she must make a change—is always the best place to begin: "I really didn't appreciate it when you lost it in the car with our friends. Yelling and carrying on like that makes me feel really tense and embarrassed. Please don't do it again." Or "Why do you withdraw from me when you're mad? It makes me feel rejected and really sad. Please don't do that anymore. Just talk to me, okay?"

Take a few minutes to think about what efforts you've made to be direct and how your efforts have been met. My clients have reported the following responses to me. Are any of these similar to the reactions you've gotten when you've shared your honest feelings?

If your partner replies with "I didn't know my anger was upsetting you so much. I will try not to raise my voice and to be calmer. Let me know how I'm doing, okay?," you probably don't need this book unless the other person just doesn't know *how* to change, in which case it will be a good guide. At least your partner is a good listener and willing to make an effort to change. But what if you get one of these all too common replies?

• *"I don't have a problem. I just get upset with what you do."* This response outright denies that anger is a problem. Angry yelling at you, ignoring you for days, or withholding affection (or many other angry faces) get relabeled: "I'm just upset." Of course the new label could be "frustrated," "annoyed," or "stressed," but they all serve to minimize the problem. Also, notice how you are blamed for your loved one's anger. What "you" do is the justification for your partner's emotional reaction, and the focus is now placed on you. The implication is that if you would only change, your partner wouldn't get "upset." So now you end up blamed for what is not really your problem to begin with. Does this sound familiar?

• *"You just want to create problems."* Another version of this one is that you enjoy/seek out the creation of problems in this relationship, whereas your partner just wants to be carefree and happy. By "constantly bringing up problems" you now have become "the problem," and if you would just relax and forget about these nonissues all would be at peace and you could spend your evenings singing "Kumbaya" together. Right? This is really crazy-making! You're living with someone who acts out anger in ways you cannot tolerate and now are told that you somehow enjoy conflict. Again, the implication of this reaction is that you must stifle your need for a change and stop making trouble for the relationship. If you would only relax and forget about these problems, they would go away. You're left with all the responsibility for making a change and will continue to be stuck with your partner's anger.

• *"Everybody gets mad. I'm just getting out my feelings, which is good."* At least there is an affirmation here that this person does get angry, but again there is no acknowledgment of your feelings and the negative impact that this anger has on the relationship. This reaction minimizes or tries to "normalize" what this person does when angry, thus making your complaint seem over the top. Also, it makes the assertion that "getting out" anger is always a good thing. Direct expression of thoughts and feelings is not only a good thing but is essential to resolving conflict in your relationship. The issue is not emotional expression but just *how* those emotions are expressed. The faces of anger shown in the box in this chapter all have one thing in common: they are ineffective and dysfunctional ways of expressing important feelings. They almost always create anguish for others and are rarely successful in accomplishing anything other than making relationship issues worse. We'll discuss many effective ways of expressing anger or other emotions in the chapters that follow.

Getting a reaction like one of these three can be frustrating, demoralizing, even disorienting. If your partner is embarrassing you with his sarcasm when you're out with friends, it's only right for him to see the light and change. If he really cared, he would, wouldn't he? If a stranger or someone with whom you have to interact only minimally acts out anger toward you in a demeaning or destructive fashion, you can walk away. You don't have to live with this person every day and put up with poorly expressed anger as a permanent fixture of your life. But getting shut down or put off by someone you love whose actions you sometimes "hate" can feel like a jail sentence with no hope of parole. You want to stay in the relationship, but what is happening is unacceptable, and you may feel you've run out of options for how to proceed.

What Options Do You Have?

Do you throw in the towel and just leave? That is not so easy to do if you love this person or have numerous bonds, like children, extended family, or financial security. Or do you just accept things as they are and cope as best you can, the "grin and bear it" solution? You wouldn't be reading this book if that were acceptable to you.

If the relationship stays as it is and you continue to be unhappy living with this person, when is it time to say "enough"? Leaving a committed relationship, particularly when children and other joint commitments tie you together may be easy for someone else to recommend, but it is never an easy decision. As we'll discuss, establishing clear boundaries for what is acceptable and what you're unwilling to tolerate is fundamental to making a decision to leave. Clearly, you would leave immediately if your safety or that of other family members were imperiled. More will be said about this sad but necessary option in Chapter 8. But first we'll explore the real possibilities that you can directly and indirectly influence what happens next with this person so that you don't have to plan an exit.

To address these issues, you need to know something about the nature of relationships: what you do can affect what the other person thinks and feels and then decides to do. The reverse is true also—what your partner does immediately impacts you and can set the stage for you to make changes you never dreamed you would make.

The Nature of Change in Relationships

How do you make someone change when this person hasn't chosen to do it on his or her own and may not even believe that a problem exists?

First, let's examine what you personally can control and the limits of your control. I'd argue that I can't control any other living thing. I cannot guilt-trip, cajole, threaten, plead, discuss, placate, or even purchase my way to getting my Burmese cat, Sy, my wife, my sons, or my clients to make changes. If another person (or cat!) is willing to listen to my needs and decides to change, then new actions are limited only by this person's basic abilities and experience. If the other person does not wish to change, I could continue to do all of these things until "blue in the face" and still be met with anger I find objectionable.

If you don't believe me, try to "make" a teenager be respectful all the time or a three-year-old stay in the backyard without building a fence. We can ask others for relief. We can reward and compliment them when they please us and even withhold or punish them in some way when they don't meet our expectations. But we are limited to persuasion and feedback—not control. And this certainly applies to the ways others we love act out their angry feelings.

There is a silver lining, however. While we can't guilt-trip or plead enough to make others stop the toxic things they are doing, we are mostly in control of what we do in response or to proactively manage living with an angry person. Once you examine what you're doing now when your loved one becomes unreasonably angry or withdrawing, you can also determine how effective that strategy has been and take steps to change it.

If Sarah decides to stop adjusting her life to her husband's intense moods, she might decide to walk away when he is getting irritable, to go places with the family even if he is "too stressed," and to stop trying to "get him to" be more relaxed (e.g., instead of not asking him to help out around the house for fear of his reaction, expect and ask him to do it). How would that change things? What new behaviors would he have to learn if she stops trying to keep his anger at bay? Would he do it?

Of course Sarah has become afraid to do these things. At almost any cost she wants to ensure that peace prevails in her home, so she adjusts to Jeff's inappropriate actions while feeling anxious about saying something to set him off. How well has her approach really worked—and at what personal cost to her?

Research into the psychology of relationships tells us that as Sarah changes in ways that don't support her husband's current behavior, he'll have to make some changes too. He will either learn to cope better or not, but Sarah will be out from under her old pattern of taking responsibility for him. She will be free to explore other options for the kind of life she wants to lead, inviting him to participate but moving forward herself nonetheless.

So how do you begin to reset your current pattern of reacting? How do you respond differently to your loved one's intense "disgust," intimidating voice, criticisms that go over the top, or stressed-out hostility? What do you do when the other person's anger is so indirect that you can't get him or her to confront the issue with you? What if you're met with shocked denial ("I don't have any issues—what is *your* problem? I'm fine!") when your loved one is withdrawing emotionally or physically or sabotaging your relationship and blaming you? Whether you're met with direct or indirect faces of anger, the chapters that follow show you the steps to learning a new pattern.

LEARNING A NEW PATTERN

It's not easy to break out of a pattern you're used to, even when you know you've gotten stuck. Psychologist Harriet Lerner describes the interdependent behaviors of a couple as a "dance." Each has "steps" that impact what the other does. Behavior patterns can become so automatic that we engage in them without being fully conscious of what we're doing. So the first step is usually to become aware of exactly how we're reacting to a loved one's "dance steps" when angry. If you don't like the current "dance," you can change the steps, and your partner will either follow your lead or not—but the old "dance of anger" is ended. In later chapters you will learn to identify what needs to be changed about your present relationship and then begin to set new expectations for what is and is not acceptable and craft a strategy for change that will embody how you will think, feel, and act differently in the future.

Taking a snapshot of the present is the first of five steps toward a new style of communication in the future. These steps are easy to remember because they correspond to the first five letters of the alphabet (A–E).

Assessing Your Relationship (A)

Chapter 2 focuses on learning how to assess your present relationship. How do you currently respond when your partner expresses anger in an unwelcome way? This first step of assessing (A) what your partner does and how you currently react is essential in deciding whether you need to try out some new approaches, whether your partner is on board or not.

If she is quite irritable and intense, do you confront your partner with the same level of intensity? Or do you try to stay out of her way? Or perhaps you bend over backward to be nice and accommodating so that your partner will have nothing to complain about? If he "switches off" when angry, how do you try to get him to talk? Do you plead for his attention or just ignore him back? Do you punish this behavior by withholding something he wants, or do you end up giving in to keep the peace? These are just a few of the possible ways you or I might respond to the faces of anger depicted in this chapter.

A questionnaire will help you evaluate the ways you've been reacting to your partner's anger. Are you happy with the current way anger unfolds, or do you need to begin to consider new ways of achieving personal and relationship goals? Your partner is fully responsible for what he does, but the reality is that he probably won't change until a change appears to be in his best interest. Your reaction certainly affects whether continuing to browbeat you, coerce you, or act out inappropriately remains in your partner's best interest. If you keep giving in, avoiding a fight at all costs, or amending your own needs and plans to avoid a controversy, in a way you've ensured that your partner's anger has paid off.

Setting New Boundaries (B)

While your partner may not wish to change or will question your rationale for change, you are now in control of what you do. First you need to consider what actions in anger are acceptable to you in the future and which are not. These become your boundaries (B), the second step toward creating change in your relationship, found in Chapter 3. Some of us do not have clearly defined boundaries for the behavior we expect from others. We may let our lives revolve around another's wants and actions and don't speak out when our own needs are being blocked or violated. This is a sad state of affairs that psychologists call "codependency." When your life and actions begin to revolve around keeping another person happy or preventing her from doing something you find unacceptable (e.g., you make excuses for your partner's outburst at a party; you give in to your partner's angry threats by avoiding your own family at Christmastime because she doesn't "like" them), you may have become a codependent. You have begun to alter your own actions to avoid upset or placate your partner to avoid the risk of an angry exchange. Soon what you need gets lost in your desire to prevent conflict; you sacrifice your own needs to ensure that your partner is calm.

The only solution is to clearly define your own boundaries: what is acceptable behavior from your partner and what is not. A personal boundary is similar to plotting a line on the ground that demarcates my property from yours. With real property, the boundary can actually be drawn on a site plan—carefully surveyed with accurate measurements. In our relationships we also need boundaries, and while we can't define them in feet or meters, we need to be clear to ourselves and others what behaviors we find acceptable and which we do not. Once you're clear about how you wish your partner to speak and act toward you, the next step is to ensure that you consistently hold to your bounds. Chapter 3 helps you define your boundaries and start sticking to them.

Changing Your Cognitions (C)

Chapter 4 examines how you have come to think about yourself and your partner and how these cognitions (C) either support your new boundaries or may be undermining them. How you think about yourself and others is what determines how you end up feeling. This is the basic premise of cognitive-behavioral therapy (CBT), a well-tested method to help people regulate their emotions and reinforce new actions. This book is based largely on the CBT approach. Chapter 4 offers many strategies to promote helpful self-talk, thinking that guides you to achieve your relationship goals. You'll acquire tools to calmly and quickly challenge and replace negative or unhelpful self-talk and immediately alter how you're feeling. By practicing these CBT ideas you will gradually alter beliefs learned early in life that have derailed you in the past.

Denial of Rewards (D)

Chapter 5 illustrates how to put your new actions into practice. First you have to avoid unwittingly paying off your partner's unwelcome expressions of anger. Called "Denial of Rewards" (D), this important step ensures that your partner gains nothing from expressing anger inappropriately. Example payoffs to avoid would be giving in to an aggressively stated demand, not speaking up for fear of intensifying your partner's loud voice, or submitting to an unreasonable request to avoid making waves. Denying your partner any rewards for her anger might mean holding your ground when met with aggressive talk, speaking up to state your opinion, and being open about your emotions, expressing them calmly and clearly. In all cases you're communicating that you and your needs matter as much as your partner's and that you will not give in to any form of angry intimidation or coercion.

Expressing Yourself Effectively (E)

You have to be able to express your ideas and needs clearly and calmly if you want your needs to be met. Rather than withholding your opinion, minimizing your feelings, or avoiding saying or doing what you need to do, you can learn to be assertive in communicating your thoughts, feelings, and needs. Good communication ends in mutual understanding and requires that both parties be willing to listen attentively and not just talk. In Chapter 5 I'll give you plenty of examples to illustrate the critical ingredients of direct communication and listening with empathy. After teaching you some practical ways of defusing your partner's anger so that it is hopefully derailed before emotions get out of control, I'll illustrate how you can resolve differences with collaboration.

Chapters 6, 7, and 8 apply what you've learned about the change process to living with four faces of intense anger: hostility, sarcasm, and verbal and physical aggression that may reach the level of abuse. For each face of anger you might be confronting with your partner, I offer concrete ideas and examples of each step you can take to dramatically improve your own experience and outcome when anger arises. Also, a no-nonsense discussion of when anger expression becomes abusive and potentially dangerous will be focused around answering the questions of when to remain and try to work things out alone or with professional help and when it is time to leave or take legal steps to ensure your own and others' safety.

Chapter 9 addresses less obvious and nuanced modes of anger expression, which can be just as destructive as their outrageous and intense brothers. I offer ideas for bringing these passive ways of communicating anger into focus to reveal underlying emotions and needs instead of continuing to sweep them under the table. You'll learn strategies for confronting denial and passive withholding of responsibility for solving relationship problems.

HOW CAN MY RELATIONSHIP CHANGE?

There's no guarantee that your partner will change. But it *is* hard for people to keep up the same old behaviors when their partner is no longer following their lead. Even if you're the only one who's made a change, the nature of the communication and behaviors between you and your partner will have changed.

When Sarah begged Jeff to get some help for his anger and stress and even suggested marital counseling, he told her he had no problems and she needed to "chill out and not get so upset about nothing." He kept playing that old song: "Yes, I get upset sometimes, but doesn't everyone? Why do you have to pick on every little thing I do? Who wouldn't be upset with their wife nagging them all the time just because they're stressed out?"

Focusing on what she could do and control (and not waiting for Jeff to see the light, over which she had no direct control), Sarah began to identify Jeff's behaviors that were unacceptable to her. We decided that she must clearly communicate immediately when his statements and behavior were becoming hostile and refuse to encourage his ire by not giving in or in any way modifying her wants and needs to accommodate his irritability. For example, she would no longer stick around and listen to his insulting litany of what was wrong with her and the kids or alter her plans based on his mood. When he handled situations calmly and effectively, she let him know how much she appreciated his efforts and tried to listen carefully to his needs as he began to be more attentive to hers. We also discussed how she could express her ideas and feelings to him while remaining calm yet being assertive and firm in holding to her new boundaries.

At first Jeff's hostility increased as he became irritated and surprised by Sarah's standing her ground, sometimes refusing to continue a conversation that was turning into shouting or critical words. Sarah found that, even when Jeff kept arguing loudly, she was in control of whether to participate and how to react. Even though Jeff didn't change right away, almost immediately Sarah felt more calm, prepared, and accepting that while she could not control his actions she sure could manage her own!

For Frank and Linda, it was important first and foremost to understand that no level of name-calling, touching, holding, restraining, or hitting was ever justified. Frank agreed with this boundary but continued to maintain that their individual actions could always be explained by what Linda did first. At first Frank refused to return to the sessions but was invited to come at any time. Linda began by setting new limits for what she would tolerate from Frank (name-calling, put-downs, and physical acting out were no longer permitted), while also agreeing that she would stop labeling her fiancé and would avoid all put-down comments and any form of physical reaction other than defending herself or leaving if the situation became dangerous. Instead, we worked on strategies to defuse the rapid escalation of aggression and to redirect her own thoughts, feelings, and actions so that resolution could be possible. We also agreed on terms for her to leave the situation to avoid further escalation and to protect her from further destructive argument. Soon Frank decided to come in to tell me "his side" of their relationship, and he too set limits for himself and for Linda. We practiced how he could react differently to ensure that the flame of anger was doused soon after igniting. Soon the couple reported that arguments were less frequent and seemed to run out of gas before escalating. In our sessions I noticed that they both were more complimentary of the other and I rarely heard the blaming and counterblaming that marked their first session.

How did they do it? They had reached a point of no return and seemed to recognize that they each had to take responsibility for themselves and make changes now or this relationship would soon be over.

When Nancy and John were not withholding and withdrawing from each other, the two reported that they had a good marriage and a lot in common. But the ways they expressed their anger created a lot of wear and tear on their relationship. I worked with each of them to set clear and realistic expectations for how they would like each other to act. Regarding anger, they were encouraged to identify early on when a discussion was becoming upsetting and then to use an "I feel" statement to communicate directly and assertively. I reviewed the destructiveness of passively expressed anger, highlighting how each partner's passive and cold approach fueled hurt and anger in the other, which was then expressed as cutting off contact. With practice they soon learned to interrupt this unseemly and unproductive pattern and instead work collaboratively to identify each other's needs and try together to get them met. Gradually they learned how to talk to each other directly and effectively instead of bailing out.

You may not be able to change your partner. But by using the many strategies you will be learning in the next chapters you can make a lot of changes to benefit yourself and, in turn, your relationship. You just might find that your partner can't help changing too.

2

RECOGNIZING HOW ANGER IS PULLING YOUR STRINGS

Think about a dance you know how to do. Maybe you learned the waltz or the two-step at a junior high dance class or recently took some salsa lessons with a friend. At first it probably felt like you and your partner had four left feet between you and moved about as smoothly as a couple of mismatched gears. Gradually you got into the swing of things, knowing that when one of you moved a leg or an arm a certain way the other should respond with a particular step, slide, or kick. Before long you found you could even have a conversation during the dance, your respective body parts seeming to do their thing without needing any explicit commands from you.

This learning capacity is great news for people who love to tango or fox-trot. It's not so great for those engaged in the dance of anger. As explained in Chapter 1, when you feel helpless to control your partner's anger, you naturally try to find some way to adapt to it. Maybe you try to minimize the stress in your partner's life or you talk and act differently to avoid inciting his ire. It wouldn't be surprising if you started to harbor a healthy dose of anger yourself. Maybe you've gotten in the habit of exacting some sort of revenge by getting in your own digs or withholding affection or fighting fire with emotional fire.

When your partner gets mad, what do you usually feel and do? You might find it a lot harder to answer that question than you would have imagined. It's kind of like giving directions to a destination you've driven to every day for the last five years. You follow the route so automatically that street names and landmarks, distances and trouble spots might be hard to conjure up. When your partner's anger has been a factor in your relationship for a significant amount of time, you've probably developed automatic, habitual responses that you're not fully aware of. In fact you might feel like you're a puppet, and it's your partner's anger that's pulling the strings.

The fact that we all react emotionally to anger, whether the other person's anger is hot and aggressive or cold and passive, makes it even harder to step back and observe ourselves. Your partner makes a snide remark, and you retaliate without thinking. Your partner yells, and you shrink and mutter an apology. Afterward, it may be hard to re-create what happened and why because your decision making wasn't necessarily cool and calculating at the time. The fact that you're reading this book tells me that the next step is not that you two kiss and make up but rather that you have an emotional response that triggers another response in this angry "action–reaction" dance in which you find yourself. And around and around the dance floor you go. Where it stops? That's the focus of this book.

There's only one way to interrupt this dysfunctional cycle, and that's to change what ***you*** *do.* But to make a helpful change, of course, you have to know what you're doing at any given time. That's the purpose of this chapter: to help you become much more aware of how you respond to your partner's anger so that you can find places to replace this particular duet with one that suits you better.

As I said in Chapter 1, you already know you have little control over what your partner does, but that doesn't mean you should be oblivious to the behaviors he or she employs to express anger. As we explore your reactions to anger, I'll help you see which faces of anger your partner wears, so you can specifically target those when we discuss each one separately later in the book.

ASSESSMENT (A): HOW DO YOU FEEL WHEN YOUR PARTNER EXPRESSES ANGER?

When there are no choices to be made, autopilot can be a boon. But inappropriate expressions of anger leave you feeling trapped, so choices are exactly what you need. You can't make them unless you can turn off autopilot and become fully present when conflict arises. "Being fully present" means being able to observe yourself more carefully so you're aware in the moment of how you are thinking, feeling, and acting. Once you're aware in this way, you can decide what you need at that moment and choose options for your reaction that are better for you and clearly set boundaries for what you will tolerate and what you will find unacceptable. Then you won't be on automatic pilot anymore, reacting so quickly and habitually that you end up feeling uncomfortable and like a pawn in your partner's anger game.

Again, you can't make your partner change just by changing how you act. But as described in Chapter 1, how you react may set the stage for your partner to try new, hopefully better, behaviors because you're no longer responding in the old ways. Your new actions disrupt your partner's well-learned habits, which won't have the effect your partner desires anymore. Most important, you end up reacting in a way that is best for *you*, a way that reduces your discomfort and helps you get your own needs met.

To help you recognize the way you think, feel, and act in response to your partner's anger, I've developed a questionnaire called the Relationship Anger Profile (RAP). This questionnaire, on pages 26–28, is informed by years of listening to clients describe the impact of anger in their lives, as well as knowledge of the common defense mechanisms observed by psychologists whenever someone feels emotionally threatened by another's behavior. It focuses on four core emotions that seem to capture the major ways we react to an angry, perhaps threatening, face of anger: anxiety, guilt, anger, and fear. Clearly these four basic emotions can't capture everything you might experience when feeling threatened by your partner's anger, but I think you'll find that they are at the core of most likely reactions to anger. You might describe yourself as "apprehensive," a form of anxiety, or you might say you felt "resentful," which is a variant of anger, for example.

Besides describing your typical emotional reactions in a variety of nuanced ways, you might be aware that you react to your partner's anger differently depending on how intense the anger gets, where you are, and who else is present. If your partner gets mad at you when you're with friends or family, you might feel so anxious or embarrassed that you think you'd do almost anything to get her to stop. If the two of you were alone at the time, you might instead react first with anger, possibly then getting fearful if your partner's anger got out of control. Or maybe your

THE RELATIONSHIP ANGER PROFILE (RAP)

Write in the name of the angry person for whom you are describing your feelings and actions: _____. Think about the last few times this person got angry and how you felt in response.

Which of the four core feelings do you experience when this person acts in an angry way toward you, whether he/she withholds what you want or withdraws in cold anger or acts sarcastic, intense, hostile, or loud/aggressive? Once you've circled Y (yes) for **one or more** emotions—anxious/tense, irritated/angry, responsible/guilty, or afraid/fearful—answer the questions that follow the ones for which you circled Y.

I feel ANXIOUS (e.g., apprehensive, worried) when this person gets mad: **Y N**. If YES, then carefully consider and answer yes or no (circle Y or N) to the following questions:

1. When I think this person might get angry, I carefully consider exactly what I am about to say before expressing it.   Y   N   [a]

2. I often find myself avoiding saying how I really feel so the other person won't get mad at me.   Y   N   [a]

3. There are certain topics I avoid if this person seems upset.   Y   N   [a]

4. Sometimes I try to change the topic or keep things from upsetting this individual (e.g., keep our children away, reduce noise, make sure everything is perfect) to avoid this person's anger.   Y   N   [b]

5. I have given in and changed my own plans or avoided going places with this person when I was concerned about an escalation of anger.   Y   N   [b]

6. I find I will avoid certain people or couples this person dislikes to avoid any possibility of anger becoming an issue.   Y   N   [b]

I feel GUILTY (e.g., responsible, sorry, apologetic) when this person gets mad: **Y N**. If YES, then carefully consider and answer yes or no (circle Y or N) to the following questions:

1. At times I find myself trying to make excuses for this person's anger—to somehow justify it to myself or others.   Y   N   [g]

2. This person can't help how angry he/she gets—it's just a personality trait that can't be changed, so I must live with it and adjust to it.   Y   N   [g]

3. When this person gets mad, it must be my fault also. It takes two to start any argument or conflict.　　Y　N　**[g]**

4. Giving in to this person is the easiest way to get the anger to stop or avoid it in the first place. Life is too short to make a big deal out of things, so I just do it his/her way to avoid the hassle of it all.　　Y　N　**[h]**

5. I try to make up for conflicts with this person by doing something nice to make him/her forget about it.　　Y　N　**[h]**

6. I know this person will get his/her way eventually, so I just don't fight it anymore. It's easier just to give in and get over my feelings.　　Y　N　**[h]**

I feel ANGRY (e.g., irritated, annoyed, enraged) when this person gets mad:　**Y　N**.　If YES, then carefully consider and answer yes or no (circle Y or N) to the following questions:

1. I spend a lot of time defending myself around this person.　　Y　N　**[c]**

2. I cannot let something this person says go if it's wrong or unfair—I feel I have to defend or justify my position.　　Y　N　**[c]**

3. I find that I am very alert to this person's negative comments about me and react to them immediately.　　Y　N　**[c]**

4. When I get mad, I sometimes do just the opposite of what this person wants, just to let him/her know that I matter too.　　Y　N　**[d]**

5. I find myself withholding what he/she wants as a kind of payback.　　Y　N　**[d]**

6. I get so mad that I sometimes stop talking or withdraw physically (e.g., leave the house, go to another room) and refuse to have anything to do with this person for hours or even days at a time.　　Y　N　**[d]**

7. When this person criticizes me, I get so annoyed I often criticize something he/she said or did in return.　　Y　N　**[e]**

cont.

THE RELATIONSHIP ANGER PROFILE (*cont.*)

8. I get very impatient and act angry myself when I am treated   Y   N   [e]
    unfairly by this person.

9. Sometimes I raise my voice in response to what this person   Y   N   [e]
    says.

10. At times I have been known to yell back at this person.   Y   N   [f]

11. When pushed to the wall, I have gotten physical with this   Y   N   [f]
    person by (one or more) blocking, pushing, holding, using
    my hands in anger, or throwing.

12. Sometimes I have said things to this person when I'm angry   Y   N   [f]
    that I would never want repeated to others I care about—it
    would embarrass me.

I feel AFRAID (e.g., fearful, terrorized) when this person gets mad: **Y   N.**   If YES,
then carefully consider and answer yes or no (circle Y or N) to the following questions:

1. When this person gets angry, I sometimes feel so fearful   Y   N   [i]
    that I am kind of paralyzed and just go along with it so it
    will stop.

2. I imagine this person will do something, whether intentional   Y   N   [i]
    or not, that results in me or someone I love (e.g., a child,
    other family member) getting hurt emotionally or physically.
    This causes me to give in.

3. I sometimes feel I cannot act or speak out for fear that the   Y   N   [i]
    situation will just get worse.

4. Sometimes I just don't know where to turn to cope with this   Y   N   [j]
    person's anger—it is so overwhelming.

5. I have thought of ending this relationship because of   Y   N   [j]
    the anger, but still care and want it to work. I feel stuck
    between the two.

6. I feel so powerless and overwhelmed at times I just shut   Y   N   [j]
    down.

partner's anger always makes you anxious and desperate to prevent it from escalating. Each emotion that's part of your reaction to your partner's anger sets the stage for some type of action on your part. Therefore, the questionnaire asks you to define how you react when experiencing one or more of the four core emotions in reaction to your partner's face(s) of anger.

Now look over your answers: Which of the core emotions did you report having? Being able to identify this emotional reaction gives you a chance to react differently, instead of immediately responding with one or more of the feelings, thoughts, or actions described below each core emotion. Look at the letter in brackets after each feeling, thought, or action for which you circled Y. Each represents an unhelpful response to the other person's anger. Write in the number of "yes" answers for each letter.

a—EDITING: _____

b—REDIRECTING/RESCHEDULING: _____

c—JUSTIFYING: _____

d—PASSIVE–AGGRESSION/WITHDRAWAL: _____

e—HOSTILITY/CRITICISM: _____

f—AGGRESSING: _____

g—RATIONALIZING: _____

h—APOLOGIZING/ATONING: _____

i—SUBJUGATING/SURRENDERING: _____

j—SHUTTING DOWN: _____

Looking at your responses, for which actions did you score at least a 1? Even a score of 1 is important as it represents an action on your part that may significantly affect how you continue to feel. To help you understand the meaning of your score on the RAP, first look at the table on the next page, which shows unhelpful reactions you just identified from the RAP to each of the core emotions when another is acting angry.

Core Emotions, Goals, and Unhelpful Reactions in Response to Your Partner's Anger

Core Emotion	Goal	Unhelpful Reactions
Anxiety	Avoiding	Editing
		Redirecting
		Rescheduling
Guilt	Atoning	Rationalizing
		Apologizing/Atoning
Anger	Defending	Justifying
	Punishing	Passive–Aggression
		Withdrawal
		Hostility/Criticism
		Aggressing
Fear	Staying Safe	Subjugating/Surrendering
		Shutting Down

WHAT DO YOU DO WHEN YOUR PARTNER GETS ANGRY?

Look over your answers to the RAP and the specific responses you've had for each core emotion. On the following pages are more detailed descriptions of unhelpful reactions to a core emotion. As you read, pay particular attention to the anger actions you've already acknowledged taking. When you've finished reading these detailed descriptions, you should have a clearer idea of which ones best describe you when you react to your partner's anger.

Anxiety

If you often respond to your partner's anger with anxiety, you might become hypervigilant to circumstances you believe set the stage for anger. When your partner begins to talk about a sensitive or emotional subject, you often tense up, preparing for anger to build. When you feel anxious, you may notice certain physical signs: your stomach may get queasy or upset; your neck, shoulders, jaw, or scalp might get tight and tense (which may lead to headaches or muscle pain); your heart may start pounding or your breathing become heavy.

These physical sensations may be triggered when your partner begins to get angry. But they can also come up even when you're just anticipating anger, such as when you think about your partner coming home from a stressful day at work, when you know you have to discuss money matters or parenting differences, or when you're wondering how to cope with an upcoming event that your partner doesn't want to attend or even discuss.

These feelings of physical discomfort are all part of the "fight-or-flight" response that's triggered whenever your body is gearing up to cope with a stressful event—in this case your partner's anger. Typical physical manifestations of anxiety are shown in more detail in the sidebar on the next page.

In fact, these symptoms occur with anxiety, anger, fear, and whenever we are just plain "stressed out"—all parts of the fight-flight response. They are important signals that not all is well and a change needs to occur: "Stop what you're doing or change what's happening!" Invariably, these symptoms mean some important need is being thwarted (your need for safety and security is threatened when your husband throws an ashtray across the room and you feel anxious or afraid, for example; we'll talk more about your needs being threatened in Chapter 3). If you experience the symptoms in the sidebar frequently, pay attention. Regularly feeling anxious or fearful in your relationship is taxing your body in ways that can cause physical/medical and emotional problems over time. Every part of your body—blood vessels, heart, muscles, gastrointestinal system, blood sugar levels, and even cholesterol—is impacted by daily stress.

Anxiety and avoidance often go hand in hand, which is understandable as a very-short-term solution: avoid the person and any situations that may lead to uncomfortable anger and you get relief. Of course short-term solutions of avoidance do not solve the problem, and you will likely

The Physiology of Anxiety: Signs and Symptoms to Look for in Yourself

Heart and blood pressure	Heart rate and blood pressure increase to supply more oxygen to brain and muscles. Pounding pulse may be observed in temples, wrists, throat, and chest. Most people cannot detect blood pressure changes, so a blood pressure cuff is necessary.
Respiration	Breathing rate will increase to get more blood to brain and muscles. Look for shallow breathing, chest heaviness, holding breath, feeling suffocated, throat feeling restricted/tight.
Gastrointestinal (GI) responses	Stomach and GI system are emptying of blood as digestion slows or halts to free up blood for brain and muscles. Look for stomach upset, queasiness, acid reflux, sometimes nausea and even vomiting, changes in bowel and urination frequency, including diarrhea and irritable bowel syndrome.
Musculoskeletal responses	All of your muscles begin to tighten, poised to help you "fight" or "flee" from the situation. Notice particularly your shoulders, neck, forehead, jaw, and also tension in your arms and legs. As arousal continues, muscle soreness or pain may result. Poor posture or improper body mechanics (e.g., sitting in a chair with inadequate back support) contributes to muscle tension and discomfort.
Vascular changes/skin temperature	Blood vessels in the face, hands, and elsewhere constrict or dilate to control blood flow. Look for the face to feel flushed, warm, or hot (described by others as "red") and the hands to feel hot with anger, cold with fear. Many notice a general flushing, like heat rising in chest and throat up to face.
Senses more acute	Vision, hearing, smell, and touch are all more sensitive and magnified. Sounds, like someone's voice, seem louder. Pupils dilate to permit better night vision, which may change focus in daytime. Movements toward you or someone touching you may seem more threatening.
Blood chemistry changes	Adrenaline and cortisol are among chemicals released into your blood to trigger the "fight-or-flight" response. Red blood cells become more "sticky" to increase your ability to clot in case you are injured. More fats and sugars are released by your liver into your blood.

face your partner's anger again and again. Did you circle "Y" for any of the following common reactions of avoidance on the RAP?

Editing

You have begun to edit what you say around this person. Melanie was in the habit of choosing her words carefully and trying to tone down her emotions so that her husband wouldn't get upset. Sometimes she would just suppress her observations about other people or the kids for fear he would overreact or start a quarrel. After a while her editing became automatic and she began to feel more removed from honest dialogue with her husband. Her true feelings and ideas were either held inside or vented with close friends or her mother. Intimacy seemed to corrode, beginning with the two of them having little "real" communication and later less physical contact, even at the lowest level, like hugging or merely touching each other.

Editing can begin almost unnoticed. You start to think about how the other person will react and adjust your words or carefully parse certain points you want to make to avoid any possibility of a confrontation. After a while **you stop thinking through your own thoughts and needs as you are so wrapped up in ensuring that this person remains calm.** You may have begun having thoughts like "It's just not worth bringing this up and starting another argument" or "If I tell him my opinion, he'll just ignore it anyway. What's the use?"

Redirecting/Rescheduling

You try to stage-manage your life to avoid possible anger episodes. Maybe when the kids start to get noisy, you shoo them into another room to play so your spouse doesn't get irritated. Or you steer your partner toward innocuous topics when the conversation starts to drift toward ones that have inflamed him in the past. Maybe you arrange your social calendar to avoid events where your partner might act irritable or withdraw or even make a scene out of anger at feeling forced to attend or to be around someone she dislikes. One of my clients would not go out to dinner with his wife and her colleagues because she made sarcastic comments and belittled him after her third glass of wine. He didn't want to embarrass both of them by calling her on it; nor did he want to humiliate her in front of her coworkers—or leave her to drive home drunk—by going home alone. He also avoided family get-togethers for fear that the critical remarks his wife made in private about his siblings would become public if she got angry at a party. His choices began revolving around his assessment of her mood and stress level. You may find yourself shielding others you care about from this unpleasantness and shielding yourself (and your partner?) from embarrassment.

Being a "traffic cop" to avoid anger incidents is effective much of the time, but you've probably begun to notice that you're turning yourself inside out at great personal cost. You may wonder when your own needs will be considered. Do you ever resent having to work so hard to keep things "normal"?

Guilt

Think for a moment about the power of guilt to motivate us to atone for some mistake we've made, particularly when we've hurt someone we love. Psychologists are kept busy around the clock helping people understand and somehow resolve their guilt over actions that may have occurred as long ago as childhood. In fact, righteous guilt is a mark of advanced civilization. It motivates us to do the right thing, to avoid hurting others, and to stay within society's boundaries. If you couldn't feel guilt, you would be much less human. People who feel little or no guilt often suffer from a condition called *antisocial personality disorder*, and they typically end up toxifying the lives of most people they touch. In fact, many end up in prison.

But how much guilt and for what? Did you actually do something with the intent or outcome of hurting or harming your partner? If so, guilt is probably appropriate. But if not, feeling guilty makes you more vulnerable to your partner's anger actions in the future. When you feel guilty (a form of anger directed at yourself), you experience immense emotional pain that you naturally want to stop. To make it stop you can either give in to your partner's demand for certain actions or take the consequences of not doing this. To make this decision you must determine what course of action is sensible and helpful given what your partner has done. When another person expresses anger toward you in an inappropriate way—such as when Nancy uses cold anger and refuses to talk to John for days at a time—feeling guilty in response and trying to atone for your "sins" is a big mistake. It will only pay off the inappropriate actions, making them more likely to recur.

Rationalizing your partner's anger actions tends to fuel and sustain these misplaced guilty feelings and may lead you to give in or atone when in fact you were the one who was wronged.

Rationalizing

This occurs when you try to talk yourself into excusing or explaining the other person's anger actions as somehow acceptable, even though at some level you know they are out of bounds. This is a thinking trick we can play on ourselves. Versions of these mental gymnastics include:

• *Stress*: "She is just so stressed that she can't help getting upset—wouldn't anyone?" Very often this plays into the hand of the angry actor because being "stressed out," "exhausted," or "just overwhelmed" are excuses at the top of the list of every angry actor I've met.

• *Legitimacy*: Here you justify being treated this way because your partner has a "good" reason to be mad. Of course anger is justifiable when an important and realistic expectation is not met (e.g., someone goes out of his way to be rude or to deprive you of something you've rightfully earned). The issue is not the anger but the mode of expressing it. Being hurtful and confrontational should not be explained away.

• *Personality*: "He's just a hot-blooded person. And he can't help it." "She has always been impatient and intense—it's just the way she is!" The justification is that being hostile or passive–aggressive is a personality trait and it is unrealistic to expect the person to change. While anger is an emotion and some of us are born with more intensity than others, this is no excuse for the poor ways we learn to express ourselves. Parents sometimes start this misconception early on in a child's life—"He's the smart one, she's the angry one," and so on—thus reinforcing a role that the child may feel she must play.

• *Stability*: "So she gets angry and we all hate it, but it is just not worth ruining a whole weekend with arguing to call her on it. Better to just keep a low profile and she'll eventually get over it. Why rock the boat?" Here, putting up with the person's anger is justified as a way of keeping the peace—at almost any price. The message the angry person gets is "I can let off some steam any way I want—no problem."

Much more will be said about the power of such thoughts to fuel unhelpful feelings and actions in Chapter 4.

Apologizing/Atoning

In contrast to merely explaining away the person's toxic actions, here you try to appease the other person by apologizing because you feel you were wrong or it's the best way to help this person stop acting angry. You might apologize for aggravating her in the first place, offering to atone for your faults in some way. For example, agreeing that your partner was "right" and you were at fault would likely end a conflict, but at what expense to your own pride and self-esteem? Clearly this is not to say that apologizing is always wrong. If you believe and the facts indicate that you violated someone's rights or wronged her in some way, apologizing can indeed be a tonic for the soul. It also helps restore the relationship to its former status. Refusing to apologize or even atone for a bad action is unlikely to resolve the rift those actions may have caused and may lead to a roadblock in reestablishing the rapport and intimacy of the relationship. Conversely, apologizing and atoning to placate a person whose anger expression was clearly inappropriate is likely to solve your problem for only a short while; it will return the next time this person doesn't get what is desired or demanded. In the long run, you have humbled yourself just to keep the peace, and this will likely lead to greater discomfort and further episodes of appeasement—clearly undermining your self-esteem and right to be heard and considered in the future.

Jared came to me having intense migraines and complaining that his relationship with Greta, his fiancée, was a major source of stress. He believed he had no choice but to constantly apologize or give in to her to stay in her good graces. He felt that if he stood up to her she would freeze him out, refusing to talk or be intimate for days at a time. So he would give in and tell her what she wanted to hear. This was not a good solution for Jared because it felt so dishonest and "wimpy" to him. He felt hurt, humiliated, and often furious with himself, but he loved Greta and did not want her to write him off as she had threatened to do many times.

Jared's migraines, for which he now took medication, had seemed to arise "suddenly" after his engagement. His neurologist suggested that he explore the stressors in his life that might be contributing to his pain. Clearly, he needed to find an alternative to constantly apologizing to Greta by standing up to her threats so the two could have an honest dialogue about their relationship. His migraines were obviously a symptom of stress caused by his unresolved needs to feel in control of his life and to feel affirmed by her.

Just leaving Greta, as his friends suggested, was not an option for Jared—he wanted to do everything he could do to make the relationship work. We implemented a treatment plan that reinforced what he was and was not willing to do to keep this relationship, as discussed in the next chapter. When his new limits were reached, Jared learned to resist apologizing, instead simply stating his own thoughts, feelings, and needs in a calm, assertive fashion. Letting the "chips fall where they may" when he honestly and directly told Greta his needs was scary to Jared at first. He was relieved to find that she did not leave him but instead began to take his feelings into account. He started to feel more confident of his worth to her and to himself.

Anger

When your partner gets angry, do you find yourself getting mad and wanting to defend yourself or lash back? Are you experiencing the symptoms of intense arousal like those on page 32? Perhaps you normally try to edit and redirect until your limit is reached; then you find yourself blowing up or paying your partner back for being unfair or hurtful. Perhaps you expect to shock your partner into being calm and caring. Or by withdrawing into "cold anger" you are "giving him some of his own medicine," a kind of tit for tat, which you believe will get him to change. Or maybe you are just so angry that you don't care what happens next. You just want to let him have it—to displace the anger you "rightly" feel onto the "cause" of your ire. Do any of the following angry reactions to anger sound like you? As you read the illustrations, think about how they've worked for you up until now.

Justifying

You can't let go of the clearly unfair things your partner says when angry. You feel you must rise to the occasion and defend each insult, misstatement, or unfair characterization even though it seems to lead to never-ending arguing. One couple I know said that each had to get in the last word, which meant that loud debates would go on for fruitless hour upon hour. Each felt completely justified in trying to win the other over, and soon they were arguing and not listening. While there is nothing wrong with calmly responding to an inaccurate point someone makes—in fact this is desirable—you must ask yourself where you cross the line into becoming so defensive and committed to winning the argument that both parties end up frustrated and angry with no resolution. Remember, the other person is already expressing a provocative face of anger. Do you find yourself taking the bait and then wishing you had stopped the discussion until tempers cooled?

Passive–Aggression/Withdrawal

You may recall from Chapter 1 that Nancy failed to clearly identify her feelings and needs through direct communication with her husband. Instead she fell back on a well-learned pattern first modeled in childhood when her father displeased her mother. Her mother would withdraw into the bedroom, refusing to talk to her husband, fix meals, or have anything to do with him until he finally apologized for his "insensitivity." Witnessing this for years, she internalized the same pattern. Nancy found herself trying to "make" John understand her justifiable hurt by punishing him in a way that he hated: she turned off and rejected him, often withdrawing to another room to dramatically illustrate her displeasure. This face of anger, meant to punish and bring about change, involved withholding what John wanted or doing the opposite of what he desired (e.g., sometimes Nancy would cook a meal John disliked when angry with him) or emotionally and even physically withdrawing (e.g., Nancy often refused sexual intimacy for days at a time to let John know how unhappy she was). Of course a major problem is that John had to guess at what Nancy's "problem" was and often would react in a similar way by withdrawing from her as a way of expressing his displeasure. Do you find yourself going to a passive face of anger to get your point across when someone you love is angry with you?

Hostility/Criticism

If you've ever stood in line with someone who was "fuming" with impatience, mumbling under his breath, and highly stressed and irritated, you know what hostility is. People who are hostile tend to be relentlessly critical when someone else fails to meet their expectations. Julie sometimes adopted a hostile face of anger with Ned in retaliation when he got impatient with her, loudly complaining that the house was "too messy" or the kids were "out of control." The more critical and loud she got, the more he would increase the intensity of his complaints, "demand-ing" that she talk with him "right now!!" As you might imagine, her "counter"-hostility only fueled more intense anger on his part, thus lead-ing to an endless loop of hostility, which only deepened the gulf between the two. Clearly, what she was doing was not working, yet Julie told me she felt locked into this vicious circle and couldn't seem to get through to her husband. When she decided to change what she did by no longer meeting his hostility with her own intense anger, the circle was broken once and for all.

Aggressing

As you will recall from Chapter 1, when anger actions are meant to hurt or harm, they become aggressive. Aggression can be expressed with hurtful words like name-calling or put-downs or of course with violent actions (any touch that is unwanted, including pushing, shoving, hit-ting, throwing, blocking, and holding). Some of my clients meet aggres-sion from their partner with counteraggression—they equal and perhaps exceed the intense and hurtful actions they're faced with. Serious conse-quences can ensue when both partners express their anger aggressively. One couple came to see me after being "thrown out" of a restaurant they enjoyed patronizing. They were told that their loud arguing and language had bothered other patrons and that it would be best if they left immediately and did not return. They were both mortified that they had been so publicly humiliated and wanted to get control of how they solved differences. As I will highlight in later chapters, alcohol tends to fuel angry acting out. While these two lacked good conflict resolution skills, it was clear that the martinis contributed to things getting out of control. As is the usual case, meeting aggressive words or actions with aggressive responses only adds fuel to the flame of anger and may lead to verbal and physical abuse. Aggression rarely solves any problem, and my clients sometimes have to experience severe consequences (like public censure, arrest, or legal punishment) to see the light. It should be noted that when a relationship becomes physically abusive, women are at least four times more likely to be injured, even if physical abuse is mutual. Much more will be said about aggression in Chapters 7 and 8: how to cope with a partner who is aggressive, when to stay, and when to leave and get help.

Elise would have an attack of gastric reflux for days following an argument with her sister. This pattern of internalizing and feeling physically sick when forced to confront family issues was "old hat" to her. Since she spent her childhood with very aggressive and controlling parents, Elise felt unentitled to express her anger to anyone and recalled getting sick and even missing school when her parents were in loud conflict. She married Ethan, who was very passive, to ensure that her life would be filled with peace. Unfortunately, his passivity often took the form of withdrawing from her and not discussing his feelings and needs when she asked for a talk. As she became frustrated and more aggressive in seeking him out and loudly demanding he respond, he withdrew more and sometimes refused to talk or retreated to his computer for hours. Never learning how to clearly express her feelings as a child, Elise would fall back on her parents' script and blow up at him, screaming, throwing things, and even pitching his computer monitor across the room on one occasion: "There. Sleep with that from now on. You obviously care more about your damned computer than me!" Countering another's destructive face of anger (such as Ethan's passive withholding and withdrawal) with your own destructive face of anger not only makes little sense but is likely to fuel the other person's actions even further. It is never justified and sets you up to be accused of being a part of the problem and not the solution (e.g., "Who are you to talk about *my* anger!")

Fear

There is a difference between feeling anxious or worried and feeling fear. Fear is your nervous system's immediate reaction to any event your brain interprets as life-threatening to you or someone you love and must protect. Fear mobilizes your body to a more extreme version of the fight-or-flight response discussed earlier and can lead to immobilization and shutting down when it escalates too far. It is kind of like a "flee" response—"This is dangerous and I feel overpowered, so let's get out of here"—but the person may not practically be able to run (e.g., he has family, work, or other responsibilities) and thus may feel stuck and overwhelmed. In essence: "I am experiencing this overwhelming internal fear but cannot mobilize myself to do anything about it." In general, more intense faces of anger like extreme hostility or verbal threats or physical aggression trigger fear for yourself or fear that others you love might be hurt emotionally or physically in some way. Your needs for safety and security are sure to be threatened, and the result is usually an intense emotional reaction. Here are some of the actions that usually come with intense fear.

Subjugating/Surrendering

Because you fear that this person might harm you or someone else you love, you may find yourself giving in and going along because you are just too frightened or immobilized to decide what you want in the situation. You're in effect surrendering your rights and responsibilities to yourself as a way of protecting yourself or others from verbal, physical, or emotional abuse. This tactic, sadly, often works to immediately shut off the other's angry tactics. By "paying off" these aversive actions by going along or giving in, you are providing powerful reinforcement for their occurrence in the future. In simple terms, we all learn from what works. In childhood we might learn that threatening to smack a kid gets us his toy truck or doll. We later learn that being a bully gets us a strange kind of respect—we are feared, so others do what we want or stay out of our way. This pattern can continue into adulthood. For example, most offices contain at least one or two "intimidators," people whose anger is so obnoxious or threatening that others go out of their way to accommodate them—when they are not trying to avoid them.

Shutting Down

While most readers of this book may not be able to relate to this reaction, it's worth noting that aggression can take a toll on the recipient's self-esteem, mood, emotions, and even health over time. I've seen individuals become so worried and/or depressed that they can't function as before. They may begin to miss social occasions, family events, work, or even retreat into using substances like alcohol or prescription drugs to get through the day. The process of shutting down occurs when one's spirit, one's individual self, is so overpowered by another's aggression and threats that it begins to retreat into dysfunction. Well before this point is reached it is imperative to get professional help and consider separating from the aggressive individual until both parties can get help to transform this sad and dysfunctional pattern.

If you see yourself engaging in one or more of the destructive behavior patterns resulting from fear, you must immediately seek advice from a professional who is familiar with these issues and can offer a plan of action to get you unstuck. As I've emphasized, **if you feel in immediate danger, take steps to protect yourself, like calling 911, leaving the situation, and alerting others.**

WHAT ARE THESE FEELINGS AND ACTIONS DOING FOR YOU?

Now that you've identified how you are reacting emotionally to your partner's anger and what actions you often take either before or after the fact, you are in a position to evaluate how you feel about what you're currently doing. Ask yourself these questions:

- How do you feel when confronted with your partner's anger? How often do you feel this way, and how are these emotional states like guilt or anxiety interfering with the quality of your day and over-all life? These are the emotional costs of the present situation.

- As you examine your anger actions described by the RAP, ask yourself:

  - Are they working to change your relationship? Do you see progress or stagnation in the ways your partner expresses anger to you?

  - Are these behaviors helping you achieve whatever your daily and longer-term goals are (e.g., a new career, providing the kind of childhood for your children you've always wanted, achieving a personal goal like having more friends or getting more fit)?

  - Do your actions fit with how you want to be as a person? Do they enhance your sense of self-respect? Would you want your son or daughter, niece or nephew to react to a boyfriend/girl-friend as you are reacting?

INCREASING SELF-AWARENESS BY STAYING PRESENT

You may already be thinking about how you'd like to change things in your relationship. Perhaps you've decided to be firmer in communicating what you want from your partner. Or you've resolved not to give in to demands made with anger, standing your ground when your needs and concerns are not being taken into account. A major goal of this book is to help you decide on new boundaries—what actions are acceptable and what are not—and to stick up for yourself when these bounds are vio-lated. But before you can try out new actions for standing up for yourself and asserting your thoughts, feelings, and needs with your partner, **you must become more aware of those moments when declaring your boundaries is necessary.**

For example, if your partner's hostile tone causes you to shrink from any confrontation and try your best not to infuriate him further by editing what you say and do, it's critical to be aware of his unpleasant tone of voice *as it begins* to intrude on your conversation. Then you can signal him early on that his manner is unacceptable. You have derailed your interaction from proceeding into the old pattern by which his hostility leads you to withdraw and give in.

In addition to being aware of how your partner is acting, it's critical to pay attention to yourself. This chapter has revealed a number of thoughts, feelings, and actions you currently experience when your partner gets mad. To make changes you must be aware of how and when these old reactions *begin* to occur so you can redirect yourself to new actions that reinforce your boundaries. For example, you can't avoid an argument with your spouse if you're not aware of saying mean things until both of you are already yelling and feeling put down. The sooner you can be aware of what your partner and you do in your angry exchange, the greater the likelihood that you can change things early on, derailing the old pattern and trying out new actions and reactions.

The table on the next page shows the external and internal events you may need to be more aware of as they occur.

Notice that the table illustrates both verbal and physical actions of your partner that may signal the onset of an anger incident. For example, are you aware that your spouse begins to get louder, becomes more emphatic with gestures like finger pointing and shaking his head "no," steps closer to you to a point where you feel intimidated or uncomfortable, or uses name-calling or insults to get your attention? These and any other actions that make you feel threatened, distressed, or uncomfortable are signals that your partner's anger expression is beginning to violate your personal boundaries.

Of course you should monitor your own self-talk, emotions, and actions too, as personal signals that the situation with your partner is becoming a problem for you and needs to be addressed. It has been noted that how you think about your partner's anger actions determines how you feel and sets the stage for what you do in response. Keeping track of your thoughts, feelings, and actions is best done by writing them down whenever your partner's anger seems "over the top." Here is a strategy that you can begin right away.

Goals of Personal Awareness

Your Partner's Actions	Your Reactions

Face(s) of Anger

Passive–aggression (e.g., withholds)

Cold anger (e.g., withdraws from you)

Sarcasm (e.g., hostile joking, snide remark)

Hostility (e.g., impatient, rude)

Aggression

   Verbal (e.g., name-calling)

   Physical (e.g., holding, restraining)

Voice Characteristics

Loudness (e.g., raising voice, "stairstepping")

Silence/"stonewalling"

Interrupting you

Tone (e.g., sharp, sarcastic)

Body Language

Facial expression (e.g., stern, pinched)

Eye contact (e.g., glaring vs. avoiding)

Physical closeness (e.g., "in your face")

Aggressive gestures (e.g., pointing finger)

Unwanted touching in any form

Thoughts that:

Fuel discomforting emotions

Reduce personal control/confidence

Rationalize partner's anger actions

Restrict your options

Feelings

Anxiety/fight-or-flight sensations

Guilt

Anger

Fear

Actions that:

Avoid communicating boundaries

Placate/reward wrong behaviors

Reduce your own sense of worth

Place you in danger

The Daily Log

Lynn decided to keep a diary of how she reacted to her boyfriend's passive–aggressive and cold angry actions when he didn't like something she did. In the past Lynn would become very solicitous (e.g., "What's wrong? What did I say now that is upsetting you? Can we talk?"). She briefly recorded the situation (e.g., what he said or did or didn't do, like talk to her) and then jotted down her thoughts, feelings, and any actions. Finally, she recorded the outcome of the encounter with him. Here is an example of one of her recordings:

> **Lynn's Daily Log Situation**: Bill stopped talking to me and went upstairs when I told him I wanted to visit with my family over Christmas break. He was clearly angry but wouldn't discuss his feelings or try to work it out.
>
> **Thoughts**: "He will never change. He clearly hates my family and will never be comfortable around them. What can I do?"
>
> **Feelings**: Sad, hopeless, and angry
>
> **Actions**: I tried to get him to talk. I went upstairs and pleaded with him to talk about this with me. He refused.
>
> **Outcome**: He won't talk, and I feel miserable. I feel completely out of control in my marriage.

This format for recording your reactions to your partner works well as it forces you to think about what happened externally (what your partner did or said) as well as how you reacted. (You'll find a blank form in the Appendix that you can photocopy if you wish.) Research on self-observation indicates that when you monitor a set of behaviors, you're more motivated and likely to alter them in the direction you desire. This effect is called *reactivity*—your actions react to your observations. As you become more aware of yourself, you can decide what and when to alter how you think, feel, and act. This sets the stage for new behavior on your part. Your behavior change then forces your partner to confront the fact that you're acting differently. What used to work to get your attention or to influence your behavior no longer works, setting the stage for your partner to make changes because sticking with old anger actions will achieve nothing and will fail to influence you! This doesn't mean your partner will be forced to change in response, but it does challenge your partner to decide whether to change or remain stuck in old actions that no longer offer him or her the same benefit.

Lynn decided to calmly inform her husband of her ideas and feelings about how they should spend their holiday. She made the case that they had not visited her family for over two years and that she believed it only fair and reasonable to be with her parents for the upcoming holidays. When he began to get angry and to raise his voice (which used to intimidate her), she calmly told him she would be happy to continue the discussion only when he spoke in a softer, calmer tone. She walked away, and soon he approached her with a calmer tone of voice—the two then worked out their differences.

I use the phrase *being present* to capture the state of heightened awareness of your partner's actions and your internal and behavioral responses as they are occurring. Being present calls on your senses to be more alert to what you are observing, hearing, and in some way feeling inside. Think about the last time you fully partook of a beautiful, sunny day. Perhaps you felt the warmth of the sun on your face, smelled the fresh air of a fall morning, heard the rustling of the wind blowing multicolored leaves through the air, and felt the first stirrings of the winter months to come.

If you now have a clearer vision of what you want to change about how you react to your partner, you must also be thinking about what actions on his or her part are unacceptable to you. What would you like this person to stop doing? How would you like to be treated from now on? This is a question that directly relates to boundaries: What will you find acceptable and not? You must decide this before you can plan for how you will react differently in the future. Chapter 3 helps you define the boundaries you wish to reinforce with new actions from now on.

3

CREATING NEW BOUNDARIES—EXPECTING NEW BEHAVIOR

Josh loves his wife, Kathy, but lately can't stand to be around her when she gets stressed out because of her senior position with a law firm. She often arrives home bristling with anger and frustration about her day, becoming loud and demanding of him and the children when things don't go as she expects. Most humiliating to Josh, she criticizes him in front of their teenagers and tunes him out when he tries to give her feedback about her out-of-control anger. Recently, she has gotten in his face and blocked him from leaving the room when all he wanted was to retreat from her nastiness. He feels extremely hurt by her remarks and is apprehensive whenever she arrives home, worrying about whether he or the kids will somehow set her off. He's at a loss for what to do, especially now that her business travel has picked up and her angry tirades just seem to be getting worse.

Jenny wants more than anything for her husband, James, to respect her. Lately, particularly when he's had a few drinks, he gets sarcastic and puts her down in front of their friends, which embarrasses her. James has threatened to separate from her more than once when he gets mad. He's so changeable that she doesn't know what to expect next from him and feels powerless to get him to calm down once he becomes upset with her. On the other hand, most of the time he is loving and a great father to their three children. She doesn't want to leave this marriage, yet she's unhappy more often than not.

When the behavior of someone we love is frustrating and confusing, we often cut the person some slack at first, even though we also feel hurt. We try to explain the behavior away; we tell ourselves it's not going to happen again; we decide to be patient and forgiving. By the time the "isolated incident" becomes a pattern, we may not know how we got where we are. This is why bringing your reactions to your partner's anger into clear focus, by using the RAP provided in Chapter 2, is such an important first step. It is not, however, enough to become fully aware of how your partner's anger makes you feel and behave. Awareness alone is a good first step, but it will not change Josh's or Jenny's situation, and it probably won't change yours either.

Josh learns from the RAP and his Daily Log that he spends much more time editing his actions to avoid Kathy's explosive anger than he would have predicted. His life revolves around coping with his anxiety and fear that she will lose it and reacting to calm her when she does lose it, which is becoming all too frequent. Jenny's responses on the RAP show that she's afraid of James and often placates him and edits what she says to avoid "making" him angrier. Bringing their reactions into focus has made it harder for Josh and Jenny to shove their discomfort into the background, and they are both coming to realize how much they want things to change.

When you establish new expectations, you're drawing boundaries, the "B" step of the A–E model. Like the lines in the center of the highway or the hedge separating two homes, boundaries clearly define a border—in this case a line between you and your partner. We all define boundaries between ourselves and others on a variety of topics, drawing lines that clearly spell out which behaviors are unacceptable to us and which are welcome. Sometimes these boundaries are explicit, while other times they are inferred by others from how we've behaved over time. While some boundaries you define between yourself and others are pretty minor, like when it's acceptable to call your house, others are of major importance, like how you wish to be treated when your partner is mad at you—for example, being told calmly how your partner feels versus being cursed at. If such boundaries are so important, how do they end up being crossed so flagrantly and so frequently? Sometimes it's because we don't realize what our boundaries are based on and therefore aren't so sure they're valid. A short course on boundaries may be helpful.

BOUNDARIES (B): A REFLECTION OF IMPORTANT PERSONAL NEEDS

When you feel frustrated, anxious, sad, angry, or even hopeless in response to your partner's anger, don't think you're alone. It's completely understandable to react when your partner acts in ways that seem to undermine the stability of your most personal and private life. If the clerk at the grocery store acts like a jerk, you may feel irritated, but you can let it go or quickly resolve your feelings by reporting him to the management. It's a limited and unimportant encounter in the larger context of your life, and it's over as quickly as it began. On the other hand, if your partner acts out anger in ways that upset you, and you don't address it, you'll continuously be faced with unpleasantness in your most important relationship.

When you feel uncomfortable with your partner's angry actions, it's because this person is integral to fulfilling your important personal needs. Uncomfortable emotions like anxiety, guilt, anger, and fear are the direct result of one or more of these needs being blocked in some way. These painful emotions have a purpose. They signal to us that we're vulnerable: someone or some situation is threatening to keep us from meeting important needs to feel safe, fulfilled, and generally happy in our daily life.

Let's look at safety. A fundamental and essential need for everyone is to feel safe and secure. Most of us would not put up with threats or verbal abuse without doing something to stop it. We'd likely call the police if faced with threats of physical harm. These reactions reflect our clear boundaries as to how we expect to be treated to feel secure and safe. When you realize that discomfort in the face of your partner's anger is a signal that your partner has violated a boundary you've set to ensure the fulfillment of an important need, it's a lot easier to stand up for your right to uphold that boundary, isn't it?

Safety, of course, isn't the only important need we share with the rest of the human race. Everyone has a unique set of needs, but on the most fundamental level there are four critical needs that every one of us must answer to live successfully. Our boundaries for ourselves and others must ensure that these needs are met.

Need 1: Security

There are two significant components to our sense of security: safety and predictability. Our brains are hardwired to keep us in a constant state of tension when we don't feel safe. We can't relax, and over time our health may be impaired. There are many things that others may say or do that can threaten our safety. For example, Jenny has begun to feel threatened by James's sudden sarcasm and irrational anger. While he has never physically harmed her, his drinking fuels a level of irritability and then intense anger that is truly scary to her at times—so unlike how her parents treated her and each other. Also, his threats to leave her and the children undermine her sense of security. Will he just leave one day? How could she cope with two young children and all their expenses? She feels paralyzed by her fears while increasingly resenting her husband's behavior. This conflict has begun to show up in her affection for him. She has buried this resentment for so long that she feels unable to discuss it, yet she is gradually withdrawing from the intimacy that she needs so badly. James interprets this reaction as her being cold and unfeeling, which is so far from the truth as to be laughable. This couple is locked in a sad vicious circle of anger actions and reactions.

Predictability is also crucial to our sense of security. In fact one of the major components of stress is uncertainty about what lies ahead. Can you trust that your basic needs will continue to be met? Can you relax into an orderly existence with your mate, family, or others? If not, you'll feel like you have to remain vigilant at all times. You may find yourself constantly on guard, checking things out to be sure you can count on your partner: Where is he going? Whom is she with? How much is he drinking? What kind of mood does she seem to be in right now? Your life circumstances can seem unpredictable when your partner, a person you depend on emotionally and practically, tends to act out emotionally, withdraws, or stops communicating directly about how he feels or what he's thinking of or preparing to do.

Josh's sense of security is threatened in a different way. Every time Kathy comes through the door after her stressful workday he worries about how tightly wound and demanding she will be. Some days she seems to manage her job with equanimity and seems happy and reasonably calm when greeting the children and telling him the story of her day. More often, though, she is loud, complaining, and hostile to Josh, as if he were to blame for her work problems. She is so unpredictable that he feels anxious every day before she comes home. Which Kathy will he see today? And what can he do "without making the situation worse" when she arrives home in a hostile, angry mood? This low sense of control he experiences greatly contributes to Josh's level of stress. Lately he's been having more headaches and tension in his neck. What to do? How to get her to understand that she is driving him away from her? How can he feel more in control of his life and his actions when the storm of anger arises?

Need 2: Affirmation

Every theory of human development describes the importance of attachment or "bonding" for us to thrive. From the time of our first interactions with our parents we need to feel affirmed as loved and respected unconditionally. If you had a warm and happy childhood with parents who were unconditionally loving, who were predictably there for you, who reacted to life's challenges in a calm manner, you may be unprepared for the intense acting out or emotional withdrawal of your partner. On the positive side, you might feel confident enough in yourself to set and enforce boundaries regarding your partner's anger.

If, on the other hand, you did not experience this loving affirmation in your own childhood, you may need a lot of affirmation from others to feel "okay" with yourself today. When your loved one withdraws, is critical or contemptuous, or withholds the intimacy you continually ask for, you may feel particularly vulnerable and threatened. In a way, these experiences mirror how you were treated by your parents. At the risk of oversimplifying a complex developmental process, this means that you may not have learned how to cope effectively with whatever emotion you experience as a result of feeling vulnerable and threatened—hurt, betrayed, frightened, or furious. You may then return to your childhood ways of reacting, whether that means switching off your own feelings, withdrawing into your room, opposing anything your partner wants, or whatever else you typically did as a child. More important, unless you've found other avenues to provide you with affirmation in your work, with other friends, in your family, or as a result of your talents, your self-esteem may be further damaged.

Having the person you love frequently act out one or more negative faces of anger can sap your confidence and rob you of the energy to carry on the relationship. Remember how hurt Josh felt whenever Kathy blew up? His need to feel affirmed by her is heightened by his childhood experience of never having felt totally acceptable to his father. Josh did well in school and was a pretty good athlete, competing on numerous teams over the years. He yearned for his dad's praise to confirm that he was proud of him. Instead, his father, having himself grown up with a strict and emotionally distant father, never learned how to be affirming. He rarely hugged Josh and was cold and reserved with Josh's mother in front of the children.

Josh's universally experienced need for affirmation was intensified as he sought clear and unambiguous expressions of love and affirmation from Kathy—his family of today. When she rejected his efforts, screamed criticisms at him, and was so angry that she would sometimes sleep in the guest room, Josh felt deep hurt along with fear that Kathy would leave him and worry that he was somehow not worthy of love. Even though Josh knew intellectually that he was a capable and competent man, these threatened inner needs for affirmation kept him unsteady and anxious much of the time in his marriage. He found himself giving in to his wife's demands and trying very hard not to anger her. He told me he would do almost anything to stop her from getting so angry. In the process he knew he was losing his own sense of identity and putting aside a lot of important personal needs in favor of pursuing affirmation from Kathy.

Despite a strong desire to change this cycle, Josh couldn't quite figure out how to do so because he blamed himself for letting his wife get under his skin and didn't understand why he did so. He had begun to view his reaction as a personal weakness, an attitude that only made it harder to figure out how to make any changes in their life together. It was therefore essential for Josh to see that a childhood marked by thwarted needs for affirmation, love, and support had left him with an increased need for the same affirmation as an adult and fewer resources for coping with the hurt he felt when faced with a hostile and rejecting partner. Once he stopped blaming himself for letting Kathy get to him, he was able to look at her actions more objectively and feel less threatened by them. He understood his own needs better and began searching for ways to get them met without depending on her "good moods," which were occurring less and less frequently. He began spending more time with his children, looked up some old friends, and joined a softball team at work—he had been quite an athlete as a teenager and had always felt good about his ability. Josh now accepted the reality that he was living with unacceptable behaviors in order to feel affirmed. He recognized that this was an understandable response given his childhood, but he could also see that it wasn't working for him. Now he could begin to confront his fears of losing Kathy and find other ways of getting his needs met.

Threats to affirmation by someone you love can be devastating and may lead to any of the unfortunate patterns of reacting described in Chapter 2, like avoiding or even getting angry yourself.

Need 3: Achievement

Once basic needs for security and affirmation are met, we are free to venture out and set and achieve personal goals. Life takes on its true spice. We may begin this journey with achievements in elementary school or in sports or the arts that cement our self-esteem as we realize the vision we have of ourselves. While experts say our self-worth should not be determined exclusively by what we achieve, can you imagine feeling really good about yourself without having some yardstick, like a job you love, children you're raising, or an organization you believe in? Research tells us that as we make things happen that we're invested in, we are happier and report feeling more fulfilled. Conversely, imagine sitting at home with no goals or few activities to invest in and continuing to feel good about yourself.

Sometimes our loved ones criticize our efforts or interfere with what we want to accomplish as a way of acting out their own anger or perhaps proving the cliché that "misery loves company" by trying to bring us down. Or maybe an angry relationship so saps our energy that our dreams begin to fade away as we just try to get through every day in the presence of a person who is hard to live with. When James feels angry and rejected by Jenny, he sometimes belittles her dreams. She's taking classes at a local community college to get a degree in social work. Jenny has always dreamed of working with abused children but instead she works part-time as a bookkeeper for a small local business to help pay the bills. Sometimes tending to the children, keeping the house going, working, and taking evening classes seems overwhelming. She wonders if she'll ever achieve her vision of a new career and feels stung by attacks from James like "Why do you persist in wasting your time and our money on an illusion? You'll never finish that program going to school two nights a week. Why kid yourself?" Jenny is very confused about where she stands with James, her career, and herself. She is starting to realize that she can't continue to live in a love–hate marriage that seems consumed by levels and expressions of anger she doesn't understand.

Need 4: Control

Over the years psychologists have studied the enormous impact of ongoing stress in our lives. What we call "stress" is actually made up of a set of bodily reactions like muscle tension, increased pulse rate, and stomach upset, along with being overly reactive to the world around us. Called the "fight-or-flight response," these reactions occur when we feel somehow overwhelmed or intimidated by too many demands, too little time, or frankly threatening events (such as yelling or threats). Anger also triggers this cascade of physiological changes. When we're stressed by life events we are much more likely to lose it. The sidebar on page 32 in Chapter 2 shows how your body reacts when anxiety, stress, or anger fuels the fight-or-flight reaction.

Research has shown that feeling in control is critical to coping with life stressors. If you're stressed out or angry and don't feel like you have options for changing things or you feel powerless to manage it, the likelihood of having emotional and health problems surges. For example, some of us feel overwhelmed by the anger of others. We might feel trapped in a relationship of cold anger—never able to resolve problems and never able to move on. Or the intensity of a partner's anger might seem so overpowering that we are stuck in quiet desperation, checkmated by anger we don't understand and seemingly cannot do anything about.

Both Josh and Jenny experience the impact that a low sense of control has on the quality of life and relationships. Josh believes he can't cope with Kathy's hostility and criticism, so he feels anxious (his chest gets tight and his heart pounds) whenever he even thinks about a confrontation with her. Lately his headaches are getting worse. Jenny has just gotten a workup by her doctor for GI problems. She often feels nauseated and has little appetite. Her physician points to stress as the culprit. She is already taking medication and has been told that she needs to get a grip on this ongoing stress or face serious health issues.

GETTING YOUR NEEDS MET IN NEW WAYS: ESTABLISHING YOUR PERSONAL BOUNDARIES

Jenny and Josh both identified important needs that helped to explain why they were each caught up in unhealthy behaviors with their angry partners. While they were often critical of themselves for "putting up with it," they now understood the reasons past and present why they felt so emotionally vulnerable. In some way they were both hesitant to risk making a change that might further upset their partner or make things even worse. Their anxiety and sometimes fear kept them locked into their old patterns of denial, placating or even giving in to their partner just to make the anger stop. Rather than blaming themselves, they now understood that these emotions grew out of the possibility of a loss: loss of a sense of security and safety, of feeling loved and affirmed, of their dreams for achievement, and of a sense of control—needs that felt threatened by their partner's inappropriate expressions of anger. Their childhood experiences made them particularly susceptible to feeling threatened when these needs were not met, and they perceived few alternatives for changing the situation without having to endure these losses. Thus they got stuck in a pattern of reacting to their partner that was painful, ineffectual, and sometimes demeaning to their self-esteem.

As they considered what new boundaries of unacceptable and acceptable behaviors they would now communicate and reinforce with their partners, Josh and Jenny both looked over a list of the types of behaviors that can block or support the fulfillment of each of the four fundamental human needs, shown in the table on the next page.

As you look over the table, ask yourself whether you see your partner as generally failing to support one or more of your important needs. If so, how? What behaviors listed in the table or others you've observed seem to block your needs? These are the behaviors that you will wish to discourage as you set new boundaries to communicate with your partner. While you probably already know how you would like your partner to respond to support your needs, look over the right column of the table for more ideas as you begin to flesh out your new boundaries.

It should be clear by now that a boundary has two components: **(1) specific unacceptable actions in words and deeds that occur when your partner is angry or otherwise upset** and **(2) desirable alternatives.**

Now that you're aware of how frequently and flagrantly some of your most fundamental needs have been thwarted by your partner's anger, you may be wondering if setting new boundaries will be a futile exercise. How do you know your partner will respond differently? How best to communicate and reinforce your boundaries so that your partner chooses to speak to you and behave toward you in acceptable ways will be explained and illustrated in detail in later chapters. For now, remem-

Partner Behaviors That Impact Your Needs

Needs	Partner Behaviors That Block Needs	Partner Behaviors That Support Needs
Safety and security	Threats Abusive words/actions Scary outbursts/rage Leaving	Calm voice/demeanor Reassurance Controlling emotions Working things out
Affirmation	Put-downs Criticism/contempt Withholding intimacy	Praising/affirming you Respect for your ideas Expressing love and care
Achievement	Discouraging remarks Withholding support Withholding resources	Encouraging you Actively contributing Helping you succeed
Personal control	Avoiding commitments Unpredictable actions Refusing to talk	Taking responsibility Being dependable/ stable Collaborating with you

ber that you can't control your partner and you can't force your partner to change. All you can focus your efforts on is your own behavior. And setting new, clear, explicit boundaries *is* a big change. In the past your partner's inappropriate expressions of anger have made you very uncomfortable at the least. Even if you knew this discomfort signaled that your needs were being denied, you probably haven't gone so far as to translate your reactions into clear, consistent definitions of what you will and will not accept from your partner. So I'll ask you to take a leap of faith and focus your attention exclusively on creating those boundaries right now without worrying about how your partner will respond. What matters first is that you assert your own needs.

The Importance of Being Specific

Think about past episodes of anger with your partner as you begin to formulate an answer to this question: **What partner words and actions** are out of bounds (unacceptable) for you in the future, and what new actions are acceptable ways of expressing anger to you? In setting a new boundary you should be as *behaviorally specific* (behaviors in word and deed) as possible. Avoid vague or ambiguous language (e.g., "bad attitude," "abusive," "obnoxious," "uncaring") when defining the boundary for your partner. Here are some examples:

> **Vague and Too General:** "In the future it is unacceptable for you to speak to me in a disrespectful way." [Does the listener really know what the speaker means by "disrespectful"?]

> **Behaviorally Specific:** "It is no longer acceptable for you to call me names, to tell me my feelings are silly, and to criticize me in front of the children."

Jenny wanted to set a boundary for James's intense anger around her. She recognized that her sense of safety and security was constantly threatened by his threats and put-downs and that giving in to him and avoiding telling him how she really felt had unwittingly reinforced his aggression and hostility, in fact making matters worse. While acknowledging she could not force him to use calm words and actions when he was frustrated by a person, like an "incompetent" clerk or waiter, or a situation, such as a shelf that wouldn't fit together as quickly as James wanted, Jenny decided that she would let him know in clear language that aggressive and hostile behavior around her was unacceptable from now on.

Keeping a Log to Focus Your Thoughts

But where to start? Sometimes people who have been tolerating undesirable behavior for a long time find themselves stymied when it comes time to get concrete about new boundaries. If the ideas in the preceding table were too general to stimulate your own ideas, you might do what helped Jenny and keep a Daily Log of your partner's anger episodes for a few weeks. This log will crystallize for you how your partner has been acting and how you have been reacting. A blank log that you can fill in is in the Appendix. Once you've filled it in for two or three weeks, look over your Daily Log and then on a separate piece of paper write down the anger behaviors that were most upsetting and unacceptable to you. For each, think about an opposite, appropriate, acceptable action you would like your partner to use to express anger or other emotions. Jenny's new boundaries are shown below.

> **Unacceptable Behaviors**: Raising his voice while standing over her, using sarcastic language; name-calling; putting her down with con-temptuous remarks, particularly in front of others; threatening to leave.

> **Acceptable Behaviors**: To use his calm words to directly express his anger and needs, to be seated when angry, to be supportive and kind in words and actions, and to confirm that together we can work it out.

Deciding on new boundaries immediately made Jenny feel more in control and assured that she had a clear set of goals: to insist in every way that these lucid and directly stated boundaries would be respected. She said it felt good to acknowledge to herself and to James that *she* could decide on what she would accept and how she would respond from now on.

Informing Your Partner of Your New Boundaries

The next step for Jenny was to inform James about her new boundar-ies. As noted earlier, we won't discuss how to assertively and directly express your thoughts and feelings until later. For many people, includ-ing Jenny, these are communication skills that have to be learned and then practiced. I'll give you an opportunity to do just that in Chapter 5. Meanwhile, the following shows the kind of exchange that often occurs once an angry person is informed that the rules have changed. (Please understand that James had never been physically aggressive or violent with Jenny. If he had been, we would have taken a different approach to communicate with him and protect Jenny, as will be discussed in Chapter 8.)

> JAMES (*coming in from work*): This place is a zoo! (*raising his voice*) What do you do all day? You're teaching our kids to be slobs like you! I've had a miserable day, and I come home to this mess! I'm out of here. (*Walks to the door, as if to leave.*)

> JENNY: Wait just a minute, James. Please sit down before you go. I want to get something off my chest. I will not take the blame

anymore for your stressful job, I will no longer stay around and listen to your loud, berating anger, and I will not be intimidated by your threats to leave me.

JAMES: What's this—are you threatening me? All I'm doing is working hard and trying to be a good husband, and now you're complaining about me? Where do you get off—I treat you wonderfully!

JENNY: That may be your opinion, but I stand by what I said. In the future, James, I expect basic courtesy from you: a calm and softer voice, even if you're mad about something, not making accusations, and expressing that you value our marriage and want to stay and work things out. If you can't do these things, I will not be available to talk or to do things with you. You have a choice, and so do I.

JAMES: We'll see. I will not be threatened by my wife or anyone else. (*Walks over to the front door, walks out, and slams it.*)

Jenny was literally shaking inside as she informed James of her boundaries. She immediately felt her old fear and apprehension that he would be intensely angry at her. She feared he might now decide to leave her, and she began to imagine how she would survive without him. In the past she would have chased after him when he left the house or repeatedly called him on his cell phone, almost begging him to be more reasonable and return home. This time we had rehearsed how she would think and what she would do to preserve her position and avoid giving in to her fears.

Upholding Your New Standards When Your Boundaries Are Violated

In most cases, announcing your new boundaries is not going to magically erase inappropriate behavior from your partner's repertoire. You also need to have a plan for reinforcing your boundaries when your partner pulls the same old tricks out of his hat. To reinforce her new boundaries with James, Jenny planned what she would do when he spoke and acted in unacceptable ways. She and I also rehearsed this new script so that she'd remember her lines when emotions began to run hot.

If James began to raise his voice, Jenny would assertively let him know that this was not acceptable around her. As soon as his voice became more intense she would calmly get his attention and ask him to please discuss the matter with a calm tone or to please stop talking or go someplace else in the house if he "had to" raise his voice. If he refused, then she would leave the situation without another word. She would not criticize him or raise her own voice to overwhelm his loudness. She would just calmly state what she needed from him (her boundary) and reinforce it by following through. She found that initially James reacted to her efforts at being assertive by stepping up the intensity of his response with statements like these:

> "Who do you think you are, telling me to be calm? I can't help it if that waiter is acting like a moron, and you should support me!"

> "You are just too sensitive. I am not raising my voice. Just making a point."

> "Go ahead! Leave if you want. Be that way, and I'll keep reacting whatever way is right for me!"

When met with hostile reactions like those of James it is important to first try to defuse the comment with one of the "defusing strategies" shown on page 100 in Chapter 5. No matter what James said to try to derail her assertion of boundaries, Jenny would use the tactic of the "broken record" to stick to her boundary and state her position once or twice: "While you certainly have a right to yell, I have a right to peace and calm as I define it when I'm around you. If you can't honor that, we can't be together right now."

When Jenny reinforced her new boundaries by altering how she reacted while continuing to state what she needed from James, she was calmly but firmly encouraging James to alter an anger pattern that had "worked" for him up until now and to communicate with her in a new, acceptable way. If he did not, she was not willing to continue to talk and do for him as if nothing was wrong. James often ended up talking to the wallpaper because he was unwilling to try to change his behavior quickly. But Jenny stayed the course, refusing to talk with him when he violated her boundary. Sometimes she "blew" it and would get drawn into his defensive retorts or into defending herself as she used to do. She would try to get back on track as soon as she found herself slipping into these old patterns. She tried to remember that behavior change occurs in a gradual way with some ups and downs. Chapter 9 discusses the roadblocks Jenny and Josh and others faced as they tried to implement the ideas in this book and how they overcame them. James finally began to get the message and talk with her more calmly since that was the only way he could express his feelings to her that she was willing to listen to. Note that Jenny did not expect her husband never to get angry but made it clear that for her there was only one way to express anger: calmly, directly, and with respect. She of course made sure she was returning the favor, communicating her anger and issues to him in the same calm and respectful way. In a way she modeled what she wanted, and this also reinforced his attempts at new anger actions.

Along similar lines, Josh decided to communicate a new boundary for Kathy after deciding that her disaffirming, loud, and demanding criticisms of him in front of the children and others had to stop. No longer at a loss for what he needed from her, he set the following boundaries:

Unacceptable Behaviors: Raising her voice, calling him names, criticizing him in front of the children, blocking him from leaving the room, and any restraint of his actions.

Acceptable Behaviors: Telling him calmly how she felt, discussing upsetting events in a normal, moderate tone of voice, asking him to step out of earshot of the children if she wished to offer constructive criticism of him, permitting him to stop the conversation and to leave to calm himself whenever he felt the need.

Notice how clear and specific Josh is in what he asks of his wife. There can be no doubt about what he expects now and in the future. Josh found a time when Kathy wasn't busy with child or household activities to sit down with her and discuss exactly how he felt about her anger expression and directly described his new boundaries. While she was speechless at first, he was pleased and surprised that she agreed with him that her anger was over the top and also told him some things that she wanted from him. Clearly he had caught her at a stress-free time (a good move on his part), when she was much more willing to listen than she would have been if she had already been irritated. They had the first real discussion about their feelings and needs in a long time, and both felt good about the conversation. Of course implementing a plan to reinforce the boundaries, similar to Jenny's strategy, was not easy and took perseverance.

FROM CHANGING THE RULES TO CHANGING YOUR THINKING

As you can see with Jenny and Josh, change is one of the hardest things to ask of anyone, and it rarely happens overnight. That's because we have to unlearn what we've learned so well. Our habits, particularly when they involve anger, seem to form easily and then stick around tenaciously. Perhaps as a self-preservation mechanism, the brain prods us to learn very carefully from any situation that threatens our basic needs. We try something out, and if we "survive," that new action becomes a stronger habit. Even if it isn't the best way to cope in the long run, we're likely to repeat it the next time we confront our partner's anger because it somehow seemed to "work." If I've learned to immediately agree with whatever my spouse wants as a way to "keep her" from getting angry at me, I have learned a new habit that "works" even if it is ruinous to my sense of self-esteem in the long run. It accomplished its short-term goal: stopping her from acting in a threatening way. This is how we learn a variety of dysfunctional behaviors that seem to stick with us, from permitting ourselves to be dominated by a friend to avoid her displeasure with us to learning to suppress our opinions at work to avoid a supervisor's wrath.

My goal is to illuminate how you can make necessary changes in how you react to your partner, as painlessly and effectively as possible given that you are up against a strong foe: your current habits in thinking and actions. By identifying how you think and replacing unhelpful self-talk with new thinking that is fact-based and affirmative, you can begin to alter how you feel when your partner gets angry. This relationship between how you think and feel now and how to alter both is described in Chapter 4. You will learn to see what your partner does through a clear lens—objectively and in a way that empowers you to feel differently: calm, optimistic, and secure in your right to be treated differently. When you don't feel anxious, guilty, angry, or afraid, you are much more likely to be able to react differently. You will no longer be a captive of your uncomfortable emotions.

4

IDENTIFYING
THE THINKING PATTERNS
THAT KEEP YOU STUCK

"There's nothing that will make Lakisha back off once she gets furious with me," says Adrian. "Every time she gets angry like that I feel really hopeless." Lakisha's way of handling her anger is to raise her voice, get right in Adrian's face, and interrupt him if he tries to explain why he did something to displease her. Her typical defense is that she has always been easy to anger but "quick to calm down." Adrian is getting tired of waiting for the calm.

As Sam starts to yell at their daughter on the way into their hotel, familiar wheels begin to spin in Sydney's head: "If I can just do a better job of controlling the kids, maybe I can keep Sam from getting so impatient with them and he won't ruin another vacation."

As usual, Charlotte has taken personal offense at Bill's attempts to bring up how their money is being spent and has retreated to the bedroom in anger. Bill has decided there's no point in continuing to try to get his wife to work with him on the bills. "Now she won't have anything to do with me for the next few days," he thinks dejectedly, "and I guess I better let her cool off and then apologize. It's the only thing that works. Meanwhile, I still don't have a clue about how we'll pay the IRS."

Adrian repeatedly feels immobilized by his fiancée's anger. Sydney keeps beating herself up for the fact that she can't seem to prevent the kids from aggravating Sam to the point where he blows up at the whole family. Bill has been on the defensive for years in the face of Charlotte's attack-and-retreat tactics. These people admit to feeling trapped. Why, then, don't they try responding differently to their partners' anger?

Adrian, Sydney, and Bill feel trapped by their partners' anger, but what really has a hold on them is their own thoughts. Adrian thinks there's no way to make Lakisha back off. Sydney thinks Sam blows up at the kids because she isn't keeping them under control. Bill thinks the only way to resolve the conflagrations set off by Charlotte's temper is to leave her alone and then apologize. These are not random ideas that each came up with out of the blue. They are well-formed perceptions reinforced by constant repetition. These ideas consistently influence how they each feel and behave when their partners get angry.

When thoughts are solidified over time, their grip is hard to break. Think about it: Tell yourself over and over that there's something scary out there in the dark and you're likely to push your fear to a panicky crescendo. Tell yourself a picture on your wall is always crooked and no amount of fiddling with it will set it straight. Tell yourself over and over that someone dislikes you and pretty soon you'll see disrespect in every innocuous gesture. Think something often enough and you're sure to end up believing it.

COGNITIONS (C):
WHAT YOU THINK IS WHAT YOU GET

Once you have assessed the way you react to your partner's anger (A—Chapter 2) and then have reviewed and set new boundaries (B—Chapter 3), you're ready to work on enforcing those boundaries. To start, you need to turn to your thinking, or cognition (C). You may be able to change your outlook and, in turn, your behavioral response to your partner's anger by examining and changing the way you think about your partner, yourself, or the situation you're faced with. Why should you do that? Because you have control only over what *you* think and do, not over what your partner thinks or does. This is where your power lies. And, as you'll see in this chapter, your thoughts are not etched in stone. *Thoughts are not facts.* You may find upon close examination, in fact, that your thoughts are faulty or at the very least exaggerated. You'll almost certainly find that they lead you nowhere but back into the trap in which you're already stuck.

When Adrian tells himself there is nothing he can do to remedy a bad situation, he is likely to feel hopeless and lose confidence in his personal power to act on his life. He lives with a sense of anxiety and dread about what he can do or stop doing to keep Lakisha from getting upset. His thinking is not about finding solutions to his problem, but only about reviewing how upsetting his fiancée's face of anger is in his life.

Starting a family vacation, Sydney feels guilty and apprehensive about how Sam will act. Her self-talk reinforces her belief that she is somehow responsible for her husband's displays of anger toward their children. Thinking this way leads her to immediately feel anxious and responsible whenever the kids start to make noise or quarrel, as children often do. Sam is a nice guy when everything goes as planned, but changes in routine like travel and holidays "stress him out," and he handles the stress poorly, reacting with irritation and volatility. Now Sydney has to act quickly to suppress the children's normal exuberance so he doesn't blow up. Notice how Sydney's self-talk not only increases her discomfort but also sets the stage for her actions (trying to keep the kids at bay to keep him calm). Looking at this situation from the outside, do you think Sydney is responsible for Sam's anger or that she can "keep him calm"? Even if you believe she can keep him calm, is the price she has to pay—sacrificing her need and right to enjoy her children to meet Sam's needs—a fair trade? As long as Sydney believes she's responsible for maintaining Sam's tranquillity, she'll keep making this inequitable bargain.

Bill's self-talk underscores his ineffectiveness in getting his partner to take joint responsibility for their finances. When Charlotte walks out on him in cold anger, leaving him to solve their problems by himself, Bill thinks he'll inevitably have to apologize to her to get the relationship back on track. He has seen the sequence of events unfold this way many times before, and he hates the feeling of rejection triggered by his wife's exits. So he is convinced that dropping the subject of contention and apologizing is the only way to lift the iron curtain. This seems fine with Charlotte, who therefore doesn't have to step up to the plate and work with her husband. As long as Bill lets his fear of rejection supersede his sense of fairness about mutual roles, he's right: nothing *will* change.

When Adrian, Sydney, and Bill look at the history of interactions involving their partners' anger, they don't see any way they could behave differently. Adrian believes he's tried "everything" and "nothing works." Sydney has a pile of evidence that the kids' boisterous behavior makes her husband mad and that when the kids are subdued, so is her husband. Bill knows Charlotte loves him and therefore believes surely she'd realize how horrible it feels to him to be shut out; the fact that she holds out till he finds the rejection unbearable convinces him that apologizing is the only way to end the standoff.

It's only natural to trust your reason the way these three do. We survive by learning from repeated observation how events, people, and environmental conditions are likely to affect each other. It makes self-preserving sense to conclude, for example, that putting your hand in a fire burns you while sitting near a fire warms you. The problem is that human volition greatly complicates matters. The fact that interactions between two people repeatedly unfold in the same way doesn't mean they *have to*, in the same way that putting your unprotected hand in the fire will inevitably scorch you. So when your partner's expression of anger always leaves you hurt and frustrated and logic tells you there's nothing else you can do, it's time to examine your beliefs about what's going on. Fortunately, cognitive scientists have discovered a way to identify how your *thinking* is keeping you stuck.

HOW WE GET TRAPPED IN OUR OWN THOUGHTS

New thinking can set the stage for feeling more optimistic and in control. Then you can plan new actions that will change the outcome of your interactions with an angry partner. But how do you know exactly what beliefs need to change?

For most of us how we think comes so naturally that it seems strange to question it at all. (Are we supposed to distrust the miraculous capacity that tells us fire burns and keeps us from singeing our hands over and over?) Our thinking feels so automatic and so much a part of us that it's hard to step back and evaluate whether it's helping or hurting us. In fact, what we *do* is so much more tangible and observable that we often focus on behavior and don't consciously realize what we're thinking at the time.

Psychologists have studied the impact of how we think and discovered that our own thoughts trap us because they can have an enormous influence over our emotions and, in turn, our behavior. They've found that depression, anxiety, fear, embarrassment, and—of particular relevance here—anger are definitely triggered by certain kinds of inaccurate thoughts to which we are all vulnerable. These thoughts take a variety of forms that we'll explore in this chapter, but because they are all inaccurate in some way, scientists call them *cognitive distortions*. These faulty ideas give rise to undesirable emotions in the same way that valid ideas lead to desirable emotions: by being part of the *self-talk*—the internal commentary, analysis, and instructions that stream through our minds during much of our waking hours—to which we are all subject.

As a simple example, let's say I tell myself that there's no way I'll ever be able to quit smoking. A quick objective analysis reveals that this thought is inaccurate: there's no way I can know for sure that I'll never be able to quit smoking. If I subscribe to this self-talk, it's likely to make me feel depressed if I want to quit, and maybe angry at myself for being "weak." It's also likely to make me give in to the urge to light another cigarette because there's not much point in trying to stop smoking if my efforts will be futile. Not only do I not end up making a change I want to make, but my self-talk becomes a self-fulfilling prophecy, which fools me into believing my thinking is accurate. This is how thoughts based on cognitive distortions reinforce negative thinking, perpetuate negative emotions, and often lead to unwise actions.

CHALLENGING OLD BELIEFS: COGNITIVE-BEHAVIORAL THERAPY

A branch of psychology called *cognitive-behavioral therapy*, or *CBT*, specifically focuses on learning how to identify and challenge these distorted thoughts so that your new thinking evokes a desirable emotion (e.g., calmness, relaxation, confidence) and helps you act in ways that serve you well. Using these CBT ideas is the best way to alter how you're thinking and over time actually change your beliefs about yourself and your relationship.

When it seems a little crazy to question our own thoughts, it's because we often confuse beliefs with facts. The belief that I'll never be able to quit smoking is not based on a fact; it's based on a cognitive distortion. But our beliefs are so deeply entrenched we may think they're as solid as facts.

Beliefs are the underlying assumptions we make about ourselves, others, and things we encounter in the world. Many of our beliefs are learned in childhood and reinforced throughout our lives. They are the filters through which we react to any situation, such as how we view good versus bad or courteous versus rude. They're hard to shake loose.

Adrian believes he's not good at handling conflict, and so he can't stand it when Lakisha (or anyone else) gets angry. This belief paralyzes him when Lakisha does get angry, as she does pretty frequently. If Adrian could change his belief to "I don't like conflict and anger but can come up with good ideas to change how I feel and react when another person gets mad," he'd free himself from his paralysis and be able to try something new with his partner. Adrian's new belief would provide him with strong reassurance that he is in control of himself and can impact his own outcomes in the future.

How do you (and Adrian) begin to adopt a new belief? *By identifying and challenging cognitive (thinking) distortions that support your old belief and replacing your self-talk with new fact-based thoughts that strengthen the new belief. By changing your actions in line with your new belief.*

Think of it as being in a debate or arguing in court against your old belief. In fact, you might view your new fact-based thoughts as "rebuttals." These rebuttals challenge the inaccuracy of the old belief. You'll find that inherent in the rebuttal or new belief is the germ of a plan to take a different kind of action. If Adrian's new belief says that he can come up with new ways to feel and react to Lakisha's anger, implicit in that belief is a plan to behave differently. As he does act in new ways that are more effective, he will further reinforce his new positive belief. Through this process Adrian is altering his thinking and his behavior—which is exactly where the term *cognitive-behavioral* comes from. Alter both at once and you begin getting new and more effective outcomes in your relationships.

To change the way you think—and, therefore, ultimately the way you feel and react to your partner's anger—you need to follow these steps:

1. Identify the unhelpful beliefs that determine how you think, feel, and act.

2. Examine these beliefs for underlying cognitive distortions that almost always reinforce unhelpful beliefs and promote uncomfortable feelings and foolish actions.

3. Formulate new beliefs based on facts that allow you to plan new actions.

Dividing this reframing into steps makes it easier to undertake this kind of change, but in reality the whole process ends up being fairly seamless. Therefore you'll find it's only natural to begin to think about new actions you might try as soon as you've come up with a new belief. In Chapter 5 we'll shift from planning new actions to taking new actions.

BELIEFS: HOW WE VIEW OURSELVES AND OUR RELATIONSHIPS

The list of unhelpful beliefs one could hold about anger and conflict in relationships is infinite. There are, however, a finite few that keep coming up in my work with clients—beliefs that often block effective communication and action with an angry partner.

Identifying Your Unhelpful Beliefs

Do any of the "Common Unhelpful Beliefs" shown in the table (left column) seem familiar? As you look over the list, identify those unhelpful beliefs that seem to agree with your own outlook on yourself and your relationship. These beliefs are reinforced every time you have a thought or engage in an action that seems to support them.

Adrian subscribed to the belief that "nothing works to get Lakisha to change" her hostility and sarcasm. He also believed that she was "incapable of changing" due to her childhood with a mother who was verbally abusive and intense. His beliefs left him few options. Since he believed that there was nothing he could do and she was not going to change by herself, he pretty much gave up and gave in to her tirades. As a result, his self-talk and his actions tended to be pessimistic and self-defeating:

***Self-talk* that was influenced by and reinforced his unhelpful beliefs:**

- "She's off on it again. I'm out of here!"

- "Why waste my breath? She just needs time to get over it, and then she'll be calm again. I'll wait her out."

- "This is just how she is. I have to suck it up, and maybe she'll change when we have kids. Meanwhile, don't stir the pot and make it worse."

Beliefs Checklist

Common Unhelpful Beliefs	Rational Beliefs
About Myself:	**About Myself:**
"I am powerless to change the situation I am in."	"I control how I feel by changing how I think and how I now choose to act."
"It's my fault when my partner gets angry."	"My partner's anger is caused by how he/she chooses to think about the situation."
"I can't handle his/her anger!"	
"I am defective [e.g., not smart enough, not skilled enough, a loser]."	"I can and will find new and effective ways of reacting."
"I am too stressed out or overwhelmed to cope."	"I am a good, but fallible, human being capable of doing what I need to do to make my life better."
"I do not deserve better treatment from my partner."	"Stress is a fact of life and no excuse not to try new coping strategies."
"I *must* have my partner's love and approval to feel okay."	"I deserve to be treated with dignity by everyone and to have my boundaries respected."
	"It is nice to be loved and receive approval but not necessary for my value as a person."
About My Partner:	**About My Partner:**
"He/she is much stronger and will overwhelm me."	"While I am powerless over my partner, I can change how I think and act, which will make life better for me."
"If I do not do what he/she expects I will be abandoned."	
"Nothing seems to work to get him/her to manage anger. This will never change—it's hopeless."	"If my partner abandons me because I stand up for my rights and boundaries, I will learn to live with it."
"My partner is abusive and may hurt me (or my children) so I better do what he/she wants."	"My partner may not change, but I can and will, and that will make my life better."

Common Unhelpful Beliefs	Rational Beliefs
About My Partner:	**About My Partner:**
"My partner is incapable of changing due to his past."	"I deserve to live in safety and to feel secure and will leave my partner if that is threatened. Giving in to abuse will only encourage it."
	"Everyone can make changes if he or she chooses to. The past is over, and what I do now determines my new future."
About the Relationship:	**About the Relationship:**
"It is a dire necessity that things remain calm at all times."	"Some conflict is inevitable between two people. It's how I handle it that determines its lasting impact on my relationship."
"I must live with things as they are—nothing will change."	
"Everyone has problems like ours—I shouldn't complain."	"Change is possible when I begin to make changes myself."
"Things will work out if I just give it enough time."	"No matter what others decide to do, I have a right to stand up for what I believe to be correct."
	"Time does not change things. New thinking and behavior changes things."

Actions that were influenced by and unwittingly also strengthened his unhelpful beliefs:

- Trying to do something nice for her to calm her down

- Carefully parsing everything he said to her to avoid any possibility of "setting her off"

- Avoiding contact with her when she was mad

Unfortunately, these thoughts and resultant actions only served to make Adrian's unhelpful beliefs seem more accurate. He would, for example, placate her, and it would seem to help calm her. His rationale was "After all, she's incapable of changing, so why not give in and get it over with?" Of course when he placated Lakisha and failed to take a stand, Lakisha was encouraged to act in this way even more.

Adrian ended up in the middle of a vicious circle: the more he gave in to Lakisha to stop her tirades (which sometimes worked), the more he believed he *should* give in, and the more he gave in, the more Lakisha was "rewarded" for her toxic actions and therefore did it all the more. His beliefs became a self-fulfilling prophecy. This of course led to more placating, and the circle continued. No wonder Adrian felt trapped and "nothing" seemed to change his dysfunctional relationship. Viewed from the outside, however, it was pretty obvious that until his beliefs, self-talk, and actions changed, he would unwittingly keep the circle spinning. Chapter 5 addresses how to limit the possibility of rewarding your partner for anger behaviors you object to and how to communicate your way to new outcomes (once your thinking changes).

Perhaps you can add to the unhelpful beliefs in the earlier table with one or two that you believe about yourself or your relationship that I omitted. The list may contain beliefs that are similar to the way you think, but it's important to have a clear understanding of your own unique, specific beliefs. So think about other ways that you see yourself, your partner, and your relationship that are unsettling and seem to be overwhelming or unmanageable.

"When my partner's anger arises, I often think that I [begin to fill in your beliefs about the impact of your partner's anger on how you think and feel about yourself and your options]

_____

_____

_____."

"When my partner gets angry, I think that he/she [begin to fill in your beliefs about how, why, and when your partner gets angry and how it impacts you]

_____

_____

_____
_____."

"When I think about how anger is expressed in this relationship, I believe that [begin to fill in your thoughts and feelings about how this relationship meets/fails to meet your expectations and how and if things can change]

_____
_____
_____."

Identifying Rational Beliefs to Substitute

Again look at the table on pages 70–71, where I've added possible Rational Beliefs as alternatives to the unhelpful beliefs listed above (see right-hand column of table).

Again, identify any of these rational beliefs that you hold. Congratulations if you've endorsed one or more of these! These beliefs support your worth as a person and your right to stand up for boundaries that help you get your own needs met. If you identified none or few of the rational beliefs, however, don't despair. Here is a strategy to begin the process of change.

First, select two or three rational beliefs you would like to strengthen (believe more firmly). You can get them from the right side of the table or come up with a positive, helpful belief on your own that will replace an unhelpful belief you checked off. Write each rational belief down on a 3" × 5" card, and on each card write out at least three positive, supportive thoughts that seem to uphold this belief. Then write out at least three new actions that would back this belief. Don't be shy—anything is possible! Here is what Adrian wrote out on his two cards:

Rational Belief: She may not change, but I can and will, and that will make my life better.

New Self-Talk to Try Out:
"I have changed many things, like when I got the job at Keatings. Even though I knew little about sales, I have done well and learned a lot."

"I am capable of almost anything I try if I put my mind to it!"

"I control what I do, and I choose to stand up for myself with Lakisha."

New Actions to Try Out:

When Lakisha raises her voice, I will keep mine level or lower it a bit.

When she demands something, I will calmly state that I will not consider her request until we can sit down and calmly discuss it. I will not give in to demands.

Keep your 3" × 5" card in your pocket, wallet, or purse and review it often as a prod to actually practice the new thinking and actions. Just stating your new belief and self-talk in your mind as often as is practical and whenever faced with provocation by your partner helps it to become stronger and more automatic.

SELF-TALK: THE INNER DIALOGUE THAT SUPPORTS YOUR BELIEFS AND DIRECTS YOUR ACTIONS

Earlier you read an example of the pessimistic, self-defeating self-talk that resulted from Adrian's belief that "nothing works to get Lakisha to change." Now you need to start uncovering your own negative self-talk to see how it reinforces your unhelpful beliefs and keeps you trapped in the same futile actions. Self-talk can be divided into three different categories:

1. **Inner comments:** These are interior observations, interpretations, and ideas about your partner, yourself, or the situation. These thoughts often arise in a stream of consciousness, and one often leads to another.
   Examples: "She is just waiting for me to give in—better get it over with!" "She loves to put me down." "Today is going to be hopeless—I know she will be out of it with her anger."

2. **Evaluations:** These are judgments about what your partner or you "should" have done or what "should" happen. Remember that these judgments are not facts but based on your own personal beliefs about the situation and may not be shared by your partner or anyone else.

Examples: "I was really foolish to get so upset." "His manners are completely lacking!" "He shouldn't have gotten so angry—for any reason!" "I'm a loser!"

3. **Self-instructions:** These are inner statements that tell you what to do or how you will feel in the future about your partner's anger actions. Self-instructions often precede external actions and sometimes can set you up to act out your own anger unhelpfully. In contrast, Dr. Donald Meichenbaum has studied the impact of what we tell ourselves to do before we do it and found that positive self-instructions about how you will react to cope with another person in the future greatly improve your success.

    Examples: "I will be furious if she again refuses to talk!" "My limit is about to be reached—then I can't be held responsible for what I do next!" "I can't take any more of his anger and yelling—I'm going to lose it myself!"

A goal of this book is to help you craft factual, helpful, and affirmative self-comments, self-evaluations, and self-instructions that strengthen your new beliefs and help you resolve differences and better communicate your needs. To make sure your self-talk supports rational, helpful beliefs, you must identify cognitive distortions that are likely to strengthen unhelpful beliefs that can keep you stuck.

Cognitive Distortions That Reinforce Unhelpful Beliefs

Look over the following, which I have culled from research into CBT and many years of surveying my clients' inner reactions to a partner's anger. For each I have provided an example or two as well as an illustration of how to immediately challenge the irrational and unhelpful thought. When one of these unhelpful thoughts arises, it's important to immediately confront the thought as what it is: a distortion—unhelpful and contributing to your problems. But identifying it as a distortion is not enough. As you will see later, you also need to counter it with a fact-based, rational thought called a *rebuttal*.

Minimizing

You tell yourself that your feelings or reactions to your partner's anger are unjustified. You convince yourself that what he or she did is just not that important.

Examples:

"I'm probably just overreacting. It isn't important enough to get him mad and ruin the rest of the day."

"If I just let it pass, it will blow over and she won't get more upset with me."

Rebuttal ideas:

"This is important and has really embarrassed me in front of our friends. I have every right to speak up and let him know this behavior is not acceptable to me."

"I cannot let it pass—she just treated me in a totally unacceptable way. If I don't let her know how I feel, she'll assume she can treat me this way in the future. If she does get upset when I speak up, I have options and can handle it."

Rationalizing

You tell yourself that there is a perfectly good explanation for your partner's angry face. You try to explain away behavior that you find toxic.

Examples:

"She is under a lot of stress and can't help it when she explodes like that. I need to be more understanding."

"I know in my heart he's a good man and would not act this way on purpose. He didn't mean what he said."

Rebuttal ideas:

"I am not a mind reader and don't know what's in her mind. I do know that her actions this evening were really hurtful to me and are unacceptable no matter how much stress she's under."

"If he wasn't a good person, I wouldn't be with him—that's not the point. His angry behavior was over the top, and that is not acceptable to me. He needs to take responsibility for what he does."

Tunnel Vision

Rather than look at the whole picture, you focus on the positive things that your partner does and quickly exclude anger actions that you don't like. You filter in what you want your partner to be like and don't look at the situation through a clear lens.

Examples:

"He *did* take us on vacation last summer, and we had a great time. He was so considerate to plan that trip."

"She is so good with the kids that I can't complain about anything. She is such a good mom."

Rebuttal ideas:

"Yes, he does do considerate things for the family, but that doesn't excuse his withdrawing from me every time he gets mad. That needs to be addressed."

"I really appreciate her parenting skills, but I also have the right to express my boundaries about what I will tolerate and what isn't acceptable."

Polarized Thinking

You see the situation through an extreme, all-or-nothing lens, which makes the situation seem overwhelming. You paint the world around you with words like *always, never, the whole situation, every, nothing.* Most things in life are painted in shades of gray, but you think in absolutes.

Examples:

"My life is *never* going to change. I feel *nothing* will get her to rein in her anger."

"The *whole* relationship is becoming hopeless. *All we ever* do is argue over the smallest thing. *Nothing* is changing, and it *never* will."

Rebuttal ideas:

"I control how I react to my life situation, and what I do next will alter my own outcomes and may encourage him to change. Regardless, I control me."

"My relationship with her is filled with a lot of wonderful times, but sometimes she loses her temper. It is those times that I need to address clearly with her and set boundaries for what I will and will not participate in."

Catastrophizing

You worry about really bad things happening, which fuels fear and may keep you from acting.

Examples:

"What if I get him so mad that he leaves me and I end up alone and unable to live any kind of decent life? I lose, and he ends up not changing anyway."

"If I confront her, she will take it out on the children. It's better that I get the brunt of her anger than harming them."

Rebuttal ideas:

"I can't predict the future. I know that his anger and withdrawal is harming me right now and I will need a plan if he threatens to leave. I can't let myself feel blackmailed into putting up with his actions."

"She loves the kids, and her harming the children is not a fact, only an unlikely possibility. I will shield the children from any discussions we have, but I must confront her on her put-downs."

Self-Deprecating

You review your own faults or limitations or negatively distort your ability, which leads to guilt or a lack of self-confidence.

Examples:

"I know I'm at fault as much as her. How can I ask her to control her anger when her blowups are caused by her frustration with me?"

"He's much better at expressing his feelings and winning an argument than I am. I get tongue-tied, and he always has an answer for anything I bring up about his anger. I just am not good at expressing myself, so why bother? It won't do any good anyway, and I'll feel even worse when he puts down what I say."

Rebuttal ideas:

"I could handle things better, but that is no excuse for her losing it and putting me down. We need to discuss our differences and work things out without yelling and name-calling. I have a right to expect that."

"So what if he is more verbally quick than I am? I need to insist that he sit down and hear me out. My ideas about how to improve our relationship are worth hearing, and I will continue to insist that they be heard and addressed."

Can you see how one or more of these distortions could end up fueling the unhelpful beliefs listed earlier in the chapter and evoking painful emotions like anxiety, sadness, or guilt that might keep you from acting to improve things? How can you give yourself permission to ask for a change in your partner's actions if your self-talk rationalizes or minimizes what he or she does? How could you successfully engage your partner in a discussion of what you think, feel, and need if your thoughts paralyze you with apprehension or outright fear of what will happen if you assert yourself?

Characteristics of Cognitive Distortions

As you looked over the unhelpful beliefs listed above and the cognitive distortions just discussed, you may have noticed a few threads that they all share. These core components of unhelpful thinking are worth remembering, even if it may be hard to remember that a particular thought you are having is *polarized thinking* or *minimizing*. What they have in common can be used as an inner "tool kit" to quickly identify and counter unhelpful self-talk before it has a chance to impair your ability to think through the situation clearly.

1. *Each is built on a premise that is not factually true.* It distorts the factual reality so that it seems overly worrisome, unsolvable, and ultimately hopeless. Each of these distortions minimizes your personal power to make changes and stand up for a position you believe in. When I was a child, I loved a police drama called *Dragnet*. Each week Sergeant Joe Friday would interview suspects and witnesses with the cautionary statement "Just the facts, ma'am! Just the facts." When the person got off track into opinions and interpretations about what happened, the indomitable Sgt. Friday would immediately (and almost endlessly) repeat that line to get the person to focus only on what was actually seen or heard and nothing else. By thinking clearly about what actually was said or done, you see the situation for what it is and nothing more. Thus the thought "I am no good at speaking up for myself" would be altered to the more factual "I don't talk as fast as my husband and often take more time to think out what I'm going to say." After all, is it "no good" to be more deliberate in thinking through what you will say, even if your partner talks faster and louder? It is a difference, purely and simply. How about the nonfactual self-talk "If I say something to her, she will blow up and I won't be able to stand it"? That can be replaced by the factual idea "She often blows up, but it isn't a fact that she will. I can stand it (I have not melted away yet) and know exactly what I want to say to her once she's calm."

2. *All cognitive distortions fail to provide any plan as to how to deal with the person or situation differently.* By just magnifying problems and failing to reinforce the reality that you can handle them in a planful way these distortions leave you kind of immobilized and frustrated with an unchanging relationship. For example:

- *Distorted self-talk*: "I know our trip will be a nightmare. He always gets so stressed out and irritable when something doesn't go right that there's bound to be a problem if we're away for two weeks."

- *Self-talk that is both factual and planful*: "The fact is I don't know exactly what will happen, but I have handled a lot worse than his angry moods in my life. If he becomes irritable, I will let him know early on that I would appreciate his either chilling out or separating from me until he's calm. If he refuses, I will separate from him for twenty or thirty minutes and check back when he's in control of himself."

You now have tools to begin to address your thinking, which is fundamental to evoking how you end up feeling and acting. You can decide whether your self-talk is similar to one or more of the cognitive distortions you've just read about. If so, you can counter your thought with one you construct by asking yourself questions that best capture the two ingredients of rational and helpful thinking:

"What are the actual facts about my partner, my own strengths, and the situation?"

"What is my plan to change how I react to my partner to better get my needs met?"

Much more will be said about how to identify and rebut unhelpful self-talk in the chapters ahead, which apply this formula to each face of anger you might confront in your relationship.

Adrian and the other people introduced at the beginning of this chapter all needed to alter how they communicated their boundaries to their partners and to ensure their actions did not unwittingly encourage or reward negative anger actions. Up until now they had acted in ways that paradoxically encouraged the very behavior they wanted to discourage, yet they didn't know exactly how to turn things around. Once you've established a new boundary and your rational thinking is supporting positive changes, you must learn and practice new behavior with your partner. If your actions don't change and support your new boundaries and beliefs, the relationship will likely stay as it is. Remember, it is what you *do*, not merely what you believe and think, that will impact your partner and your own outcomes most. Chapter 5 provides you with ideas for fulfilling steps D (Denial of Rewards) and E (Effective Expression of New Boundaries) of the A–E change model to help you fulfill your new goals.

5

TAKING NEW ACTIONS
AND GETTING
BETTER OUTCOMES

Cara knew she had to do something different to get her husband's attention. Sean's irritability and hostility had reached a point where she found herself thinking of leaving him. "Why stay in this hopeless situation?" she asked me. "I've told him he needs to get help with his constant 'stress' and moodiness. Lately his negativity and anger are over the top. He yells and curses at drivers, he is demanding and impatient with service people when we go out, and he can't seem to shake off any situation that doesn't go 'right' in his opinion. Sometimes he gets so close to my face it's scary."

No wonder Cara feels helpless. Despite her repeated requests that Sean get help, she is faced with a husband who doesn't seem to think he has a problem. Why can't he see that his anger is triggered more easily every day? It's as if they're living in parallel worlds, and Cara is losing hope that they'll ever be able to meet in the middle. As you know from the preceding chapters, however, there are ways to get off that track and back onto a road that leads where you want to go. They start with going back to the beginning and assessing the problem objectively and systematically (A in our model for change).

When Cara completed the RAP in Chapter 2, she recognized that her role in the couple's dance of anger had not been limited to pointing out the problem to Sean and suggesting he seek help in solving it. Despite desperately wanting him to change, she had been unwittingly rewarding him for *not* changing. Over and over she had acceded to his requests and edited most of what she thought and did around her husband as a way of keeping the peace. Cara cringed when she remembered how she had told her sister and brother-in-law not to come over for Thanksgiving dinner because Sean couldn't stand their children's noise and "unruly, bratty" behavior. How guilty she had felt making that call, and afterward how resentful that her family would not be a part of their holiday. But at the time she couldn't bear the idea that she would probably "set Sean off" if she confronted his "selfishness" in keeping her from her sister on what was usually an occasion to share with loved ones.

Filling out the RAP also showed Cara how often she rationalized giving in to Sean's moods and demands on the theory that he would eventually realize he had a problem with his anger and change. Seeing how much time had passed without any positive change motivated Cara to try to set new boundaries (B). This was difficult for her since her behavioral patterns had become deeply ingrained. So Cara used the Daily Log in Chapter 2 to observe her husband's anger episodes and her own responses and ended up able to articulate boundaries that she felt were reasonable for Sean's actions. She tried to make them as behaviorally specific as possible so both she and Sean would be crystal clear as to whether they were being met.

Cara understood that she wouldn't be ready to explain her new boundaries to Sean until her objectives were fleshed out and clear. In the past she had tried to get through to Sean mainly by pointing out what she disliked about his angry actions. She hadn't realized until recently that she rarely articulated what new actions she wanted instead. So, for each unacceptable behavior, she crafted a goal for the behavior she expected from him. Each acceptable behavior was worded as specifically as possible. Saying she was looking for an "improved attitude" or wanted to be "treated with respect" would get her nowhere, as she had discovered so often in the past. These vague demands only gave Sean an escape hatch, and he would quickly brush off her complaints again. Instead, she paired each complaint with a specific behavior goal and also told him what she would do when she noticed that he was violating her new boundaries.

SETTING SPECIFIC NEW BOUNDARIES FOR SPECIFIC COMPLAINTS

- *Unacceptable:* Raising his voice; yelling at her and others.
- *Acceptable:* To express his opinions, feelings, and needs

using a calm tone of voice, the way he would talk to a client or colleague at work. If Sean started raising his voice, Cara would extend her palm in a "stop" gesture with the phrase "Excuse me?" This was a clear cue to Sean to either lower his voice or risk her halting the conversation.

- *Unacceptable:* Getting in Cara's face.
- *Acceptable:* When provoked, Sean would stay at least the length of her arm away from her (easy to measure by her extending her arm outward). If Sean got too close, Cara would immediately extend her arm and ask him to back away.

- *Unacceptable:* Calling anyone names (e.g., "idiots," "morons," or, his favorite, "incompetents"), including Cara and the children.
- *Acceptable:* Sean would talk about others by describing their behaviors and his thoughts and feelings about them. He would refer to others by their given name when known and not with a pejorative label (e.g., "butthead," "Miss Priss").

- *Unacceptable:* Harsh criticism, defined as making critical and demeaning comments (e.g., "He can't string five words together coherently" and "She is a waste of my time!").
- *Acceptable:* To speak about others' perceived flaws by focusing on behavior and offering specific ideas for constructive resolution (e.g., "I would appreciate your focusing on one topic at a time" or "I have little in common with her and would like not to invite them over again"). He would try to say something positive to balance a negative remark whenever possible (e.g., "I know that you are really trying hard to keep this house neat and together. Could you please buy a magazine rack for the living room so we can keep newspapers and magazines off the coffee table and chairs?").

ENFORCING NEW BOUNDARIES WITH THE HELP OF NEW BELIEFS

As you know from Chapter 4, it's difficult to enforce new boundaries when your old beliefs are telling you it's okay to stay in the rut you've been stuck in. When Cara reviewed her beliefs about herself, Sean, and anger, she was able to challenge a number of unhelpful cognitions/thinking (C). She practiced thinking affirming thoughts about herself and immediately challenging cognitive distortions that had been strengthening her self-deprecating and disabling beliefs. These are some of the unhelpful beliefs she confronted:

Unhelpful Belief: "If I create stress for Sean, it is my fault if he gets mad."

New Belief to Reinforce in Thoughts and Actions: "Sean is totally responsible for how he feels. His stress is determined by his thinking, not by what I do."

Supportive Self-Talk: "I will stay focused on doing what I think is best for me and my family, no matter how mad or stressed out Sean gets. He can have input when he is calm and kind to us."

Unhelpful Belief: "My relationship with Sean is hopeless. He will never change, and I must live with him as he is."

New Belief to Reinforce in Thoughts and Actions: "I determine what is acceptable to me, not Sean. If I change what I do, the relationship will change because I will feel better, regardless of what Sean chooses to do."

Supportive Self-Talk: "I can and will stay the course of my new boundaries. Sean will change or not, but I will feel better and have more of the life I need to have."

Looking over the "Beliefs Checklist" table in Chapter 4, Cara realized she had come to believe she was powerless over the situation—nothing she could do would "work" to change Sean's behavior. This belief and her self-talk—like "Why try to talk to him? It will accomplish nothing and only set him off" and "He can't help how he is. His parents are just like him, so just live with it!"—included a lot of forecasting, catastrophizing, and minimizing of her own strengths. She seemed locked into a pattern where the more he acted out of control, the more she gave in and avoided any confrontation. Enacting this pattern fueled more depression and hopelessness and further negative thinking, which then reinforced her sense of despair and the futility of making any changes in her life.

COMMUNICATING NEW BOUNDARIES—
AND NEW WAYS OF REACTING
WHEN THEY ARE VIOLATED

Changing her boundaries and thinking involved important personal change and new awareness on Cara's part. Without these internal changes, Cara wouldn't be able to bow out of the dance of anger with her husband. But these inner changes would not impact Sean until Cara's outward behavior changed to match them.

Cara approached this next step with the greatest trepidation of all. How could she possibly reinforce her new boundaries and stick to her guns with her husband when he had virtually ignored everything she'd said about his anger in the past? Not only had he completely disregarded her complaints about the way he expressed his anger, he often took them as an opportunity to turn her statements around and blame her: "If you would be more organized and competent in running this house, I wouldn't get so upset. You're the one with the problem. I'm just trying to make a living for us and don't need any lectures from you." Sean was an attorney and particularly adept at arguing his point of view. Cara would end up feeling not only dejected that she couldn't seem to get through to him but also hurt by his counterattack. Usually she gave up and withdrew from him until he "apologized," as she called it. "I guess I blew it," he'd say. "I was just under a lot of stress and lost it. If I hurt your feelings, I'm sorry, but you've got to realize how hard it is to deal with my job."

With the heightened awareness that Cara was developing, she started to notice that Sean's apologies were almost always empty gestures: "*If* I did something wrong, then I apologize." Sean was always kinder to her for a few days after Cara accepted his "apology," but now she saw this as mere feeble gestures. She realized now that she had been selling herself short by taking his excuses as a sign of true remorse.

Cara was tired of that merry-go-round and wanted to learn effective ways of communicating her new boundaries to her husband that would deny him any payoff. She didn't want to accede to his self-centered wishes just to avoid his anger. She no longer wanted him to think he could keep indulging himself in inappropriate anger as long as he uttered a few brief apologies he didn't seem to mean. She wanted to learn to inform him effectively of exactly what she needed and expected in the future. And she wanted to be armed with effective ways to respond when he violated her new boundaries, as well as ways to reinforce any positive efforts he made. After all, she still loved her husband and wanted their marriage to endure: she didn't want to be purely confrontational but also encouraging whenever there was any chance to do so.

NO GAIN BUT PAIN: DENIAL OF REWARDS (D) FOR ANGRY ACTIONS

Cara's attempts to get her husband to seek help for his inappropriate expressions of anger failed not because she was a terrible communicator, as she feared, but because her messages were mixed. She'd tell Sean he was out of control and needed to do something about it, but then she'd inadvertently reward him for the way he acted when angry. She'd orchestrate their lives to avoid stressing him out, which only told him it was okay for him to lose it whenever he did feel stress. She'd accept the apologies delivered with that all-powerful "if," which only told him he got to be the one to decide if and when she was hurt, and to use his excuse that his job was hard, which meant as long as he was working he was justified in blowing up at will. Now that she had set new boundaries and embraced new beliefs, she needed to deny her husband the rewards she had been providing for his angry actions (D in your new model for dealing with a partner's anger).

Since the beginning of this book, I've been emphasizing the critical point that you are powerless to make your partner do anything, just as Cara was powerless to get her husband to seek help just because she told him he should. You can only decide what you will do differently to better get your needs met and to ensure a safe and calm living environment for yourself and your family. **Denial of rewards is the only exception to this rule.** Through extensive study of how we learn and unlearn behaviors, psychologists have discovered certain principles that suggest that the only way you can have a direct impact on whether your partner changes is to **make sure that he or she receives no reward or other positive outcome for noxious or toxic anger actions.** This means that your partner does not get what he or she wants or achieve a personal goal or purpose by acting inappropriately angry around you.

Want Your Partner to Stop Repeating Behavior You Don't Like? Stop Rewarding That Behavior

Here's how this works:

If your reaction—not discussing your own needs, carefully editing what you say, doing what your partner wants without disagreement—fulfills or achieves your partner's objectives, *he or she will do it more often in the future.*

If your reaction to your partner fails to fulfill or achieve your partner's objectives, *he or she will likely do it less often in the future.* Its strength as a habit is reduced.

Your reaction right now doesn't guarantee that your partner will stop this instance of the undesirable behavior right now. No action of yours has the power to control another person like a robot moved by a remote control. But it *can* influence what happens in the long run: **The outcome of an action— either positive or negative—determines whether it is strengthened or weakened in the future.**

Possible Payoffs from Typical Reactions to Anger

Editing

In limiting your discussions and stated expectations with your partner to those you perceive will be less likely to elicit anger, you stifle your own needs and limit possible solutions to relationship issues.

Possible positive outcomes for your partner:

- Your partner avoids discussing a topic perceived as unpleasant.

- You rarely discuss your own opinions and needs, which paves the way for your partner to do what he or she wants with little conflict or respect for your needs.

- You encourage a relationship where problems don't get discussed or resolved (forcing you to "live with it," encouraging the status quo), which your partner may seek.

Redirecting/Rescheduling

In stage-managing your life to reduce stress for your partner (so he or she doesn't get angry), you avoid events or activities that you or others, such as your children, might enjoy.

Possible positive outcomes for your partner:

- Your partner avoids doing anything he or she perceives as undesirable or stressful, even if you find the activity desirable. Family gatherings, friendships, or activities you might enjoy are curtailed or avoided altogether so that your partner's needs come first and everyone else's needs come second.

- Your partner is in control of what you do, whom you see, and where you go. This gives your partner immense power over you.

Rationalizing

When you excuse or explain away your partner's angry actions to yourself or others, you lose any sense of entitlement to a calm, safe, rational environment that meets your own needs. You may even feel guilty if you think angry thoughts about what your partner does.

Possible positive outcomes for your partner:

- By not being held accountable for his or her actions, your partner gets off the hook and is greatly encouraged to behave in a self-aggrandizing, self-satisfying way that disregards your (unstated) feelings in the future.

- You play into the self-centered thinking of your partner, justifying and strengthening his or her current angry actions by making excuses for this behavior.

Apologizing/Atoning

By apologizing and appeasing your partner as a way to get him or her to treat you better, you let your own needs fall by the wayside and place yourself in a one-down position.

Possible positive outcomes for your partner:

- You further justify your partner's inappropriate actions and remove any motivation for your partner to change.

- You place yourself in a demeaning position of weakness that gives you no platform from which to protest when your partner does something hurtful. You increase his or her power by admitting to being wrong when you objectively know you're not.

Justifying/Passive–Aggression/Hostility/Criticism

When you show one or more of these faces of anger, you have become defensive or angry in a way that is uncomfortable for you and may feed into more conflict. Your own arousal negatively affects every part of your body, leading to intense stress, bodily symptoms (tight muscles, stomach symptoms, headaches, etc.), and sometimes health problems. Eating yourself up with anger or getting into a fight with your partner rarely resolves the problems you face and only fuels more discomfort for you.

Possible positive outcomes for your partner:

- Your clear anger and upset may be perceived as a victory—you are now as miserable as your partner. And being drawn into an angry argument leaves you no closer to getting your own needs met; you only end up with the empty postargument feeling of regret or resentment that continues to eat at you. If your partner wants to punish you in some way, he or she has certainly succeeded.

- Your partner feels justified because "You clearly have a problem with your anger *too*!!!" You must now justify why you get "just as mad" as your partner. Even if you point to the fact that your partner "started it," your partner is likely to view it as a lame explanation for why you acted in the same way you wish your partner wouldn't act—and deep down you'll probably agree. In my experience, those with anger problems often want to normalize and explain away their own anger by rationalizing: "I am no more angry than others/my wife/my boss, etc." When you engage in a negative face of anger, you play into this rationalization.

Subjugating/Surrendering/Shutting Down

Giving in or giving up or just withdrawing inside when you're frightened of what your partner will say or do is an immediate way to cope. You attempt to avoid all risk of angering your partner by trying to disappear—just giving your partner what he or she wants and becoming kind of invisible. You lose any sense of identity and self-esteem when this becomes your way of coping. As I said earlier, if you are fearful, you must seek help and possibly leave home and seek safety.

Possible positive outcomes for your partner:

- Your partner gets to have total power over you: your mind, actions, and spirit. This is never okay, although if your partner has been diagnosed with a mental illness or painful medical problem, you may mistakenly believe you're obligated to make allowances. Turning inward in that case is not helping your partner; it's enabling inappropriate behavior. More is said about this issue in Chapters 7 and 8, where abuse in relationships is discussed.

- Your partner gets to do whatever he or she wants with no conflict or interference from you. You have become a vessel to carry out your partner's wishes and little more. You may be a "maid," "nanny," "waiter," "cook," "sexual partner," or "breadwinner," but you have little significance other than meeting your partner's needs.

- When and how to encourage your partner to seek professional assistance can be tricky if your partner does not recognize this problem or discounts the need to get help. A discussion of these issues is found in Chapter 6. Excellent resources for health issues you may encounter that exacerbate anger are included in the Suggested Resources at the back of the book.

If you have gotten this far in this book, you obviously want to find a way to preserve your relationship, if at all possible, but live within it differently. To define new expectations for your partner's behavior, you must communicate your needs in a way that denies your partner any rewards for poor behavior like those just discussed. Fortunately, this form of clear, effective communication has been well studied. Learning its components is the final step in changing the dance of anger with your partner.

EFFECTIVE EXPRESSION OF BOUNDARIES (E): CLEARLY COMMUNICATING YOUR NEEDS

Cara knew that she tended to edit her thoughts, feelings, needs, and actions to avoid "stressing" Sean and making him mad. She often redirected her children or altered her plans to avoid people, places, and things that would aggravate him, and she resented how much she had stifled herself just to keep him somewhat calm. Cara decided to stop these patterns of reacting immediately, instead reinforcing her own needs in a calm, caring, but firm way that would no longer encourage Sean's outbursts. To deny him any rewards for his anger actions, she would start reacting in these ways:

Instead of prophesying what would make him mad and avoiding these activities/situations, Cara would assertively communicate her boundaries by telling him exactly what she **thought** and **felt** and **needed** from him and for herself and not take responsibility for how Sean might react. She would no longer curtail or revise her plans just because they might stress him out. Instead she would express herself clearly and then invite him to provide input about how he felt and what he wanted to happen so they could decide together what to do and where to go. If he began getting upset, she would communicate her boundaries in no uncertain terms and let him know she would not continue the conversation if they could not calmly talk and decide together. Sean would therefore no longer get any positive outcome from raising his voice, name-calling, and demanding. He would have to discuss *with* her, not talk *to* her.

This, of course, is always easier said than done. Cara wasn't sure she could stick to this plan without caving in to her husband. It was clear to me that she needed a new way to express herself that would decrease the likelihood of conflict with Sean. I explained that most research and clinical experience has endorsed a mode of clear, direct, and easy-to-learn communication for couples that sharply defines the roles of each party:

Sender (speaker): Communicates personal awareness—thoughts, feelings, and needs—in a direct, behaviorally specific manner with words, actions, and tone of voice.

Receiver (listener): Actively listens to the sender/speaker, trying to figure out how the other person thinks and feels and what he or she wants and needs to happen. The receiver/listener focuses attention on the sender/speaker with eye contact and body position, does not interrupt, and occasionally paraphrases what the other person is communicating.

Once the receiver indicates to the sender's satisfaction that the message has been heard accurately (the receiver paraphrases what was heard, and the sender acknowledges whether it is accurate), the roles reverse and the receiver takes the floor to share his or her personal awareness about the issue in the same way that the sender has.

This process made sense to Cara, but she was understandably worried about her ability to draw Sean into active listening without instigating more conflict. So we broke down the two-way communication process into the following components:

Preparation

We can all relate to running afoul of ourselves in communicating with our partners, friends, or family. Maybe we were too blunt or aggressive or just too "wishy-washy." Whatever our gaffe may have been, we probably felt we had not put our best foot forward and then had to explain or reexplain what we meant. I have certainly put my foot in my mouth when talking about an important personal matter and regretted not having spent some time thinking through what I wanted to communicate before beginning to speak. By then all you can do is try to repair the damage.

Preparation to communicate means you are well aware of what you want to communicate and how you wish to do it to maximize the likelihood that you will be listened to. Good communication according to most communication theorists means that the receiver has accurately heard what the sender wished to convey. Therefore, just talking to your partner, even if your words are well reasoned and stated calmly, is not good communication. It is talking, not communicating. Perhaps you can relate to what this feels like: you earnestly try to convey your issues to your partner, and it feels like he or she doesn't get it, interrupts you, or talks about him- or herself with no sign that you were heard. Pretty frustrating, isn't it?

Cara had certainly been there. So to prepare for what she hoped would be a better attempt at getting through to Sean, she focused on her awareness of *herself, where and when* she communicated, and how to assess *how upset* Sean was before deciding to go ahead with what she wanted to say using these guidelines.

Awareness of Self

Regardless of what the issue is (an example for Cara was how Sean treated her in front of her friends), you must first be aware of your thoughts and ideas, your feelings, and what you want to happen (your boundaries) to satisfy the needs for safety/security, affirmation, achievement, and control in the future discussed in Chapter 3. *You are not ready to communicate until you've figured this out.*

Awareness of Context

Finding the right time and place to communicate this awareness to your partner is essential to reduce distractions and discomfort. In general, you should avoid situations where what you're doing—driving a car, eating in a restaurant, shopping at a mall—will likely distract your partner from listening and may add stress for both of you. Most important is to avoid embarrassing your partner by offering feedback in the presence of others. I have often worked with angry patients who were confronted about their anger by their partners when good friends, parents, or other family members were present and were so "humiliated" that they felt compelled to be defensive and "attack back." The last thing you want when expressing important needs is to instigate defensiveness, which will surely block listening to you and perhaps fuel an argument.

Awareness of Your Partner's Arousal Level

No, you can't read your partner's mind to find out exactly how your partner is feeling when you decide to communicate, but by now you are probably aware of the external signs that strongly suggest the internal building of emotion. Your partner's *arousal level*—the degree to which he or she is physiologically prepared to fight or flee, an automatic response described in Chapter 2—plays a tremendous role in how your partner is likely to perceive and react to your heartfelt statement of your boundaries and needs. Recall the last times this person was clearly angry and aroused. What did you notice in your partner's facial expression, tone of voice, body position, and movements, as well as the content of his or her communications, right before and during the anger episode? The table on the facing page lists some common signs that your partner's arousal may be increasing, indicating that this is not a good time to communicate your position. If your partner always seems to act in these ways

Common External Signs of Anger Arousal

Partner Actions and Words	Signs to Look For
Facial Expression	• Face flushed due to blood vessels vasodilating. • Staring or glaring at you. Pupils dilated. Or absence of eye contact. • Shaking head "no" as you talk.
Body Position/ Movements	• Stepping into your space/getting too close. • Pacing. • Choppy/aggressive hand/arm movements. Pointing finger at you. • Any form of touching you when angry, even if not hurtful (e.g., holding you back, finger poking, blocking your path). • Leaving situation. Not facing you/turning away.
Voice Tone and Manner	• Raising voice. Yelling to make a point. Or speaking in an unusually low tone. • Laughing when obviously angry/sarcastic tone. • Stonewalling (refusing to talk). Minimal responses, like "Whatever!" and "Right!" • Interrupting you.
Content of Statements	• Cursing of any kind. • Very hurtful criticism of you or your personal traits. • Name-calling or using inflammatory words about you or others. • Immediately blaming you. • Defensiveness ("You do it also," "NO," "Never," "Not me," etc.) • Changing the subject.

when you try to talk, you need to employ one or more defusing strategies like those you will find later in this chapter.

While the signs listed in the table provide useful hints for what to look for, your past experience with your partner is probably your best guide to when he or she is becoming aroused. Finding another time to talk when you feel strongly about an issue may be frustrating for you, but pursuing a discussion with a partner who is physiologically aroused to anger is generally fruitless and will likely lead to an argument or worse. At higher levels of arousal your partner's ability to focus and hear what you're saying is compromised. Even worse, arousal makes it harder to put on the brakes and inhibit expressions of anger.

Equally important is ensuring that your own level of anger arousal is not elevated before you begin this discussion for the same reasons. Recognizing the feeling of anger early on gives your partner and you a better chance of managing it, as I detailed in my previous book, *Taking Charge of Anger*. Meanwhile, though, you can be aware of five factors that always have an impact on anger arousal. If you know any of the five *S*'s described below is currently a problem for you or your partner, you should tread with caution and consider finding a better time to talk about your feelings.

1. *Sleep*: When you've had insufficient sleep, less than seven to eight hours for most adults, you're less able to carry out any task, much less communicate intense feelings in an incendiary situation. This means if you're not getting to sleep, staying asleep, and awakening in a manner that leaves you feeling refreshed in the morning, your attempts to communicate calmly with your spouse may be fruitless. Likewise, if your partner hasn't been sleeping well, this may not be a good time to try to talk. Some medications, activity late in the evening, gastrointestinal problems, anxiety, and clinical depression are among the factors that can cause problems with good sleep habits. If you or your partner has chronic problems getting a good night's sleep, you might want to explore these possible causes with your physician, who may order further sleep studies to determine a treatment plan.

2. *Stress*: Changes and adaptations (a new job, a new boss, holiday travel, etc.), as well as perceived threats, cause stress. If you notice the symptoms of physiological arousal reviewed in Chapter 2, if you tend to worry or dread upcoming situations or can't put problems out of your

mind, you may find yourself less able to cope with emotional situations in a measured way. The same is true for your partner.

3. *Sustenance*: When you (or your partner) haven't eaten nutritiously or often enough, you may notice irritability increasing.

4. *Substances*: Alcohol in any quantity, but surely when overdone, can diminish the ability to inhibit words and actions. In general, avoid any discussion of contentious personal feelings and needs when either of you is consuming alcoholic beverages. Wait for a time when both of you can think clearly. Interestingly, about sixty-five percent of couple/family violence occurs when one or both parties are drinking.

5. *Sickness*: If you or your partner is ill, in pain, or otherwise uncomfortable due to some form of acute illness (such as a bad cold or flu) or chronic illness (migraine headaches, lower back problems, etc.), it's going to be harder to tolerate stress and inhibit high emotion and inappropriate actions.

Memorize the five *S*'s so you can use this information to assess yourself and your partner before deciding to embark on a serious, emotion-laden talk about your relationship or to expose yourself to a stressful situation that may explode. If your partner tends to show more intense faces of anger, this advice is particularly germane and may avoid placing you in situations that could be threatening or outright dangerous. To learn more about the five *S*'s, see *Taking Charge of Anger* (see Suggested Resources).

Using the "I" Message: Conveying Your Personal Boundaries

Once you've found a good time and context to express yourself, I recommend using a well-known method called the "I" message to discuss what you know best: your own thoughts, feelings, and needs—that is, your boundaries: how you wish to be treated in the future. Instead of blaming or accusing your partner with statements like "You're selfish" and "You don't care about anyone but yourself," which only fuel rebuttals and defensiveness, the idea is to speak in a personal way about how the situation has affected you and what you would like your partner to do differently. An "I" message has these components, as illustrated by how Cara decided to approach Sean:

Describe the Situation Factually

"Sean, last night when I suggested we visit my parents, you told me *you were too stressed out and refused to go.* Your voice was *loud,* and you *didn't permit any discussion* about it. Also, you may not be aware of it, but you were so close to my face—about a foot away—that I felt intimidated and will not permit that ever again. You called my parents names, as you often do, like 'slobs,' 'child-like,' and 'meddlers.' You also called me 'selfish' and a 'weak loser.'" Even though Cara must use the word *you* to objectively describe what happened, she just describes Sean's actions and her feelings and needs without resorting to name-calling or mind-reading Sean's values or motives ("You only care about yourself," "You couldn't care less about my feelings!") or blaming him.

Tell Your Thoughts, Ideas, and Opinions

"In my opinion *we should be able to talk out how we both feel about my parents and decide together* when to visit. I also think that we *need to see them* at least once a month and go with a *relaxed and positive* attitude."

Tell Your Feelings

"Sean, when you got so mad and said those things to me, I felt very *hurt* and *discouraged.* I also felt *embarrassed* that the children overheard you yelling at me."

Tell What You Need

This is where you describe your new boundary in behavioral terms, as Cara did: "In the future I need for you to sit down and calmly listen to my requests to have contact with my parents. Please keep your voice low, just like you would talk with a colleague at work. When you get in my face, it's scary and I don't like it. Please stay at least an arm's length away from me when we discuss an emotional issue. In the future, do not use name-calling, like 'moron,' or 'incompetent,' to refer to me or anyone. And be willing to problem-solve with me when would be a good time to visit."

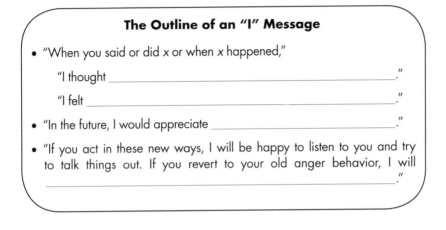

The Outline of an "I" Message

- "When you said or did x or when x happened,"

  "I thought _____."

  "I felt _____."

- "In the future, I would appreciate _____."

- "If you act in these new ways, I will be happy to listen to you and try to talk things out. If you revert to your old anger behavior, I will _____."

Describe Future Outcomes

"If you talk with me in these new ways in the future, I will be happy to listen in return and try to work things out with you. If you revert to your old anger behaviors, I will immediately end the conversation and make my own plans."

Turnabout Is Only Fair: Actively Listening to Your Partner

Listening may feel like a lost art in a culture that seems to value yelling and interrupting each other on news programs and talk shows. Deborah Tannen, a well-known linguist, called this the "argument culture" in her 1999 book with the same name. It almost seems like the goal is to make sure your opinion is the loudest and most forcefully presented. In fact, without good listening effective communication cannot occur. If Sean turns away and pays little or no attention to what Cara says, no matter how effectively she uses the "I" form of communication, he is unlikely to understand her position and needs. Unless Sean understands how upsetting his anger actions have been and knows what her boundaries are, he will have little reason to change. So, how does she make him see the light—how does she get him to pay close attention to her heartfelt expression?

By expressing her awareness in a nonthreatening manner using the "I" message, Cara reduces the likelihood of escalating the interaction and roadblocking Sean's listening to her. She sticks to factual events as she saw them and does not attack him in any way. While he might disagree with her view of things, she has not raised the ante with provocative language or intense rhetoric.

Also, if she actively invites his calm response ("Sean, could you respond to what I just said and asked for?") and listens to him no matter how self-serving his answer might seem, she encourages him to talk and not escalate his anger. She models the behavior she would like from him as the conversation continues. If Sean yelled at her or called her names and Cara immediately yelled back and justified herself with "You do it too!" Cara could be accused of being hypocritical, and her message would be diluted by her actions. Instead, Cara embodies in her listening the behaviors of active concern and empathy that she would like from Sean. You can do the same with your partner, starting with focusing exclusively on the conversation, stopping any competing activities like watching TV, reading, and fiddling with a PDA so you can give your partner your full attention following the guidelines for "active listening" on the facing page.

Defusing Provocation

Sometimes, no matter how hard you try to be direct and calm in using your "I" message approach, your partner makes things difficult. He or she might try to change the topic, get loud and abusive, or even become threatening. In all cases you can end the talk by calling a "STOP" as I discussed in *Taking Charge of Anger*. This and other strategies for defusing a difficult conversation are found below.

Defusing Another's Angry Face

• **Calm clarifying.** Ask other for **more information**—gives you time to dampen arousal and plan a strategy.

"It would really help if you could tell me exactly what you mean by my being 'selfish' and exactly when you think I am."

• **Mirroring. Repeat back** the essence of what the other said so he or she can hear your impact.

"What I hear you saying is that you think I never call Mom and Dad and that you carry the entire load of caring for them. Is that right?"

• **Content-to-process shift.** Ask the other for a pause so you can

A Primer for Active Listening

Mode of Communication	The Behaviors of Listening to Your Partner
	Body Language
Facial Expression	• Look directly at partner with reasonable eye contact without staring or glaring. • Show facial interest. • Try to keep face relaxed and smile when appropriate. • Turn your body toward partner.
Body Position	• Sit down if possible and invite partner to sit. • Lean forward a bit. • Avoid distracting hand and body movements (e.g., twiddling fingers, biting nails, shaking leg). • Keep arms uncrossed.
Gestures and Movement	• Nod your head when you agree or to show interest.
	Voice Style
Volume and Tone	• Even if your partner begins to raise his/her voice, keep your voice level. • Avoid any sarcasm/edge. • Avoid "stony" silence.
Encouragers	• Use minimal, soft encouragement for partner efforts at talking (e.g., "Yes, I understand," "Mm hmm").
	Content of Responses
Reflecting Back Feelings	• Listen for how partner is feeling and acknowledge feelings ("Sounds like you're pretty angry"; "I hear your sadness").
Paraphrasing or Summarizing Key Points	• Acknowledge his/her ideas, needs, or thoughts (e.g., "So you want me to avoid confronting you in front of our friends? Is that right?" "You think we should visit Mom for Thanksgiving this year and my parents next?")

both **discuss how the conversation could be improved**—focus on the process of how you are communicating. May need some **ground rules**.

> "It feels like we are getting off the topic and this is getting intense. What if we talk about how we can discuss this issue better? I would suggest that I listen to you for as long as it takes to get out your ideas, then you listen to my points the same way. And that we try to keep our voices calm. What do you think would help us stay on track?"

- **Agreement in fact or principle.**
    - **Agree** quickly with anything you can agree with to "take the wind" out of the other's sails.

> "You know, I agree with what you said. I do not spend enough time with Mom and Dad."

    - **Agree in principle**. While not agreeing with the specific allegation someone makes, agree with the principle behind it.

> "While I don't agree that I 'never' call Mom and Dad, let's not quibble over that. I do agree with your main point that we should try to do more for them. I intend to try."

- **Avoiding "stairstepping."** When the other gets louder, don't escalate, but instead stay level or even **bring your voice lower**, down the "stairs" of intensity.

- **Model a relaxed posture.** Utilize the impact of body position and gestures on how another reacts to you.

    - **Invite the other to be seated** if you are both standing. Immediately this reduces physiological tension. If the other refuses, you sit and use a conditional suggestion: "I really want to hear what you have to say but wish you would sit so I can relax and just listen."
    - **Lean back** and try to **breathe more slowly** and rhythmically and the other is very likely to copy ("pace") what you do.
    - Make your **gestures more smooth and relaxed** and, as you **look at the other,** show interest.

- **The "broken record."** When you are making a reasonable request, continue to **calmly repeat your request** until the other hears you. This works if you are patient in most circumstances. If not, use a STOP phrase (see below).

> "I really do intend to call our parents more often."

> "As I said, I will call them, perhaps this weekend."

> "When I call them, as I've agreed, I know we will both feel better about it."

• **Suggest a "STOP" if you feel threatened or very angry or the conversation is going nowhere.** Let the other know that you need to take a break to think things over. Make it clear that **this is not negotiable**.

> "This discussion feels really intense, and I think we need to pause for a while to collect our thoughts. I will seek you out later on to see when we can arrange to continue."

Rehearsals: Practice Makes Perfect

Cara's anxiety about Sean's possible reactions "that might last for days" seemed to overshadow her desire for change. I decided she needed to practice with me or someone she trusted using these new communication strategies so they would start to become automatic and easy to access. New behavior must be practiced to become habitual. Practice can take two forms:

Cognitive Rehearsal

You vividly picture in your mind a situation involving your partner and see yourself reacting in new and desirable ways to reinforce your boundaries. It helps to imagine that your partner responds in ways that are hard to deal with so you can think about and practice in imagination how to react when the going gets tough. Just practicing everything going smoothly is easier but does not prepare you for challenging eventualities. How can imagining your reactions impact your actual reactions when faced with your partner? Think about all the times in your life that you thought through what you would say or do before you actually did it: in school, speaking in public, or prior to resolving a problem with a friend or family member. It's human nature to rethink how we'll react before the fact. Research and my clinical experience tell me that cognitive rehearsals create a kind of inner map to guide you when you actually face a challenge. Also, they help to reduce your anxiety, worries, or outright fear about confronting your partner. By doing something we fear, in imagination or reality, we expose ourselves to our worst-case possibilities, and this weakens our fear. This is the way CBT therapists treat anxiety and fear every day. The more you assert yourself with your partner in fact or imagination, the easier it is to do it automatically. You're building new habits and extinguishing your worries each time you practice assertive communication with your partner.

Behavioral Rehearsal

In this type of rehearsal you practice your new ways of communicating your ideas, feelings, and needs with a trusted friend or therapist. Every time you actually make an effort to talk things out differently with your partner counts as a behavioral rehearsal too. If using a practice partner, you instruct that person to act in some of the ways your real partner acts so you can practice your new ways of reacting. Practice in a mock situation can give you the freedom to learn new skills gradually, rather than trying to acquire them in the heat of the moment with your partner. It also gives you a chance to get feedback from your rehearsal partner as to how you did.

Cara began rehearsing by vividly imagining how she would talk with Sean about what she wanted using the "I" message approach. We discussed any problems she felt she might encounter, such as Sean's possible objections to what she planned to say and how she might defuse any sign of Sean's anger as she spoke, and she incorporated these ideas into how she imagined herself responding. Then I behaviorally rehearsed with her what she had already practiced imaginably. I played the part of Sean, and she practiced expressing her new boundaries as I tried different ways of reacting for her to practice responding to. By the time we were done, she felt much more confident that she could confront him in these new ways and that there was a good chance he might listen to her. Most important, her anxiety about talking out her feelings and needs had dissipated a lot, and she was now willing to talk with him directly.

APPLYING THE BASICS:
FROM "A TO E" TO REAL LIFE

You have now been introduced to all the components involved in turning your life with your partner in a new direction. You have access to the basic tools and strategies you'll need to decide how you would like your relationship to change. You've learned to assess how your partner's expression of anger is affecting you emotionally and how you've been reacting to these episodes. You may have already decided whether your current approach has been in your best interest. If not, you've seen examples of how others have crafted new boundaries for anger behaviors they are no longer willing to accept, as well as deciding on the new behaviors they want to encourage in the future. Perhaps you're already thinking of the new boundaries you want to communicate and reinforce in your own life. These boundaries can be enforced in new, consistent ways only if your thinking matches these goals. So you've learned to identify beliefs and self-talk that detract from your confidence and must be replaced with objective and helpful thinking that will make you feel secure and committed to standing up for yourself.

You also know now that there is only one way you have the power to impact your partner's behavior, and that's by denying your partner any rewards for the angry behavior you find intolerable. So that you can make your new boundaries stick, you've learned the "I" form of assertive communication as well as listening skills that ensure your discussions with your partner are successful in communicating how you think and feel and what you want for your future, while staying on track and minimizing the likelihood of an unhelpful argument.

Practicing with your new tools and strategies will increase your chances of successfully communicating and enforcing the new boundaries that can protect you from your partner's anger. But it's not easy, as you know, to put into effect skills that you've learned only in rehearsals. The more you know about how to deal with your partner's chosen faces of anger, the better prepared you'll be to communicate your needs and expectations and avoid getting embroiled in even more conflict. Each of the next chapters goes into one of those faces of anger in more depth, showing how you can apply the A–E model you've been reading about to a particular mode of intense/active anger or passive–indirect anger expression. You'll get more ideas for surmounting roadblocks through the stories of others like you. Whether your partner chooses to change or not, the changes you make in yourself will surely transform your personal life for the better.

PART II

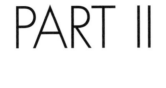

Overcoming the Different "Faces" of Anger

6

LOUD, IMPATIENT,
AND "OVER THE TOP"
Confronting Hostility

Jack was a senior executive with a major telecommunications company who seemed obsessed with doing things faster, more efficiently, and more "intelligently." At work his employees feared his blowups, which could be triggered whenever Jack was "disappointed" in the effort, speed, or efficiency with which tasks were completed. His wife, Pamela, described a family vacation when Jack treated packing as a timed task. When their children were taking too long to pack and the family couldn't leave precisely at 9:00 A.M. (a time that Jack, for some reason known only to Jack, had set), he blew up, cursing, loudly complaining, pacing, and muttering under his breath. Jack often set these kinds of unrealistic expectations, like assuming his children would be ready to leave on a family holiday at 9:00 A.M., when the family had never been able to get up, dress, eat breakfast, and pack before 11:00. Jack's expectations set him up for an angry outburst that put a damper on the family's enjoyment and created problems in his relationship with Pamela, who refused to talk to him for the first few hours of their trip.

Jack's impatience and free-floating anger with any person or situation that did not measure up to his standards was becoming a frequent unwelcome visitor to Pamela's life. I call the kind of intense, irritable expression of impatience and anger demonstrated by Jack *hostility*. In those whose anger has a face like Jack's, it's very common for people to set themselves up for their own explosion. Onlookers nervously stand by knowing the eruption is inevitable but that its onset will be unpredictable. The only thing they feel sure of is that it will likely leave a lot of devastation in its wake—like an active volcano towering over a town like Pompeii. When the eruption does occur, a vacation is ruined, a pall descends over an entire office, plans disintegrate, and everyone in the vicinity is forced to regroup.

Hostile people like Jack aren't aiming to hurt anyone, even though their expression of anger often does hurt or harm others. *Hostility* is a diffuse, intense emotional state that may in any given situation end up directed toward things—the Internet service that "always goes down," the traffic that "gets worse every day," even the "stupid newspaper" that the paperboy seems to throw purposely right where someone can trip over it—but not intentionally at another person. Anger expressed through cutting words—name-calling or put-downs—or actions like pushing, slapping, or hitting, with the intent to hurt or harm another person, is what we call *aggression*. Hostility clearly lacks the focus of aggression.

> **Hostility** is a kind of free-floating anger that has no clear human object but can be aroused by any situation that fails to meet the angry person's expectations. This venting or display of intense anger is often related to high levels of stress in the person's life.

Jack often ended up apologizing for his intensity, and his insistence that he didn't mean to hurt others or make them uncomfortable was clearly sincere. With professional treatment Jack learned to accept that, harmful intent or not, his hostile behavior was often toxic and unacceptable to the people he cared about most. It needed to be managed.

Does your partner's anger usually take the shape of hostility? Would you describe him as someone who has a short fuse? Would you say she is tightly wound and sets "crazy" standards in an apparent attempt to control her environment, only to end up furious when those standards aren't met? Does your partner seem stressed out by this constant tension between how he or she expects the world to function and how it behaves in reality? If so, this chapter will offer you some tips for confronting the face of anger that keeps you on edge, dreading the next explosion. Keep in mind, however, that many people who struggle with anger express it in more than one way. Therefore, you'll probably benefit from reading the rest of the chapters to get an idea of whether your partner expresses anger in other inappropriate ways and to learn how to deal with them too.

Rita was a good friend and a great partner to Jocelyn. She was talented, funny, and quick with the right comment or comedic view of life just when Jocelyn needed it most. She was everything Jocelyn could want in a life partnership. Theirs had lasted many years, through good times and bad. Still, Jocelyn was thinking of leaving Rita because of the "twenty percent" of the time that she felt "swamped" by her partner's intense anger. Rita would frequently come home from work filled with outrage over clients who were "impossible" and a boss she couldn't stand. Unfortunately, this rage too often spilled over into her personal life. Jocelyn repeatedly felt like a hostage to Rita's diatribes about the many people who let her down. Rita, it turns out, was a demanding perfectionist, a characteristic that Jocelyn admired in many ways. Though quite financially successful in her position with a brokerage firm, Rita could be described as "suffering fools" poorly. When her anger was aroused, she was never abusive or demeaning to Jocelyn. But when life did not go her way, Rita could be expected to make a scene with assorted wait staff in restaurants, most store clerks, and all drivers who failed to meet Rita's high and immutable expectations. Rita's favorite word was *should*, as in "He should turn in his license he is so incompetent!" and "You shouldn't have purchased that TV without checking more websites" and "She should be fired!"

Jocelyn often felt anxious and wary around Rita: When would she explode and at what or whom? Would an evening of dinner and theater devolve into Rita being impatient with everyone or telling off the maître d'? Rita's unpredictable emotional purges had become intolerable to Jocelyn, and yet she loved her partner and wanted very much for the relationship to go on. Just reasoning with Rita (for the umpteenth time) had not resulted in any quelling of her intensity. By now Jocelyn was feeling resigned to a choice between living in a threatening and emotionally intense world or leaving. She saw few options in between.

Bill and Jasmine had been together for about three years when they both sought help in coping with what they called "conflict" and "poor communication." Jasmine admitted she had known that Bill had a short fuse from the first weeks of their relationship, but she had overlooked his volatility and intensity in the interest of making him happy and keeping things stable. She described herself as the calming peacemaker, and both she and Bill described him as prone to temper outbursts, particularly related to time and "competence" issues. The couple had three young children. Jasmine was concerned that Bill's anger style would be transmitted to the kids. She also feared any changes or sudden upsets that might trigger Bill's hostility. Those triggers ranged from someone disappointing him to a clerk he designated incompetent to an unthinking friend or anyone else who failed to come through as Bill expected. And the list seemed to keep growing.

If you think you may be living with a Jack, Rita, or Bill, take a closer look at your partner to be sure hostility is the best definition of your partner's anger. Each of the hostile individuals you just met display many characteristics of a personality type that has been linked to coronary artery disease: the so-called "Type A" personality described by Drs. Rosenman and Friedman in 1974. Does your partner have any of the following characteristics?

• *Time impatience.* This means living as if in a race with time. Is your partner impatient with himself or others if things are not done quickly (or "competently") enough? Does she show signs of irritation and agitation when waiting for someone else, constantly looking at her watch, and demanding to know "When are we leaving?!"?

• *Polyphasic behavior.* This means trying to do two or three things at the same time to be overly "efficient." Rosenman and Friedman once described a heart patient who would try to exercise on his treadmill, balance his checkbook, and watch the news all at the same time. This multitasking effort is inherently stressful and raises physiological arousal, setting the stage for a blowup. Does your partner set himself up like this?

• *Free-floating hostility.* Because of its very nature, it's hard to put your finger on free-floating hostility. But it's characterized by being quickly aroused physiologically, which is translated into bitter, critical, or pessimistic comments, agitation, and a general demeanor of disgust or disapproval. Where others might appear to shrug off mundane disappointments, overlook the typical shortcomings we all exhibit, and be reasonably optimistic, the Type A personality is often disgruntled, picky, and dissatisfied. This component of the Type A style in particular is the focus of this chapter; it's also apparently the most damaging component to the health of the Type A person. Researcher Redford Williams has studied the impact of Type A on health and finds that hostility is the component that is most responsible for cardiac problems and has a debilitating effect on overall health.

WHEN TENSION AND UPSET ARE CONSTANT VISITORS: IS YOUR PARTNER HOSTILE?

What is it like living with a hostile/intense partner? How is your life in the relationship impacted? That's the important question for you to answer in this and the next chapters: How is my partner's face of anger affecting my life and the life of our relationship? When you can answer this question, you are well on your way to knowing how you want your relationship to change for the better. Answering this question is the assessment (A) part of the A–E model. Your assessment of how your partner's anger is affecting you will help you redraw your boundaries (B), adopt new beliefs and other thoughts, or cognitions (C), that will help you pursue your goals with your partner, and then deny your partner any rewards for continuing to express anger in inappropriate ways (D) while expressing yourself effectively (E) when your standards are violated.

Do you see your partner and you in any of the following descriptions?

- *"He is never satisfied. No one ever seems to meet his expectations!"* Pamela often felt it was impossible to live up to Jack's demands for how things "should" be done. He always seemed to be disappointed or let down by family, friends, and the many people who sold, served, repaired, or delivered the "things" in his life. He could even have an outburst when the TV went on the blink or the computer refused to comply with a keystroke. Pamela recalled Jack throwing his cell phone across the room when it failed to function properly. When Pamela reacted with condemnation for his "child-like display" in front of the children, Jack countered (as he often did) by blaming. "If this phone had been manufactured properly, this wouldn't have happened," he shouted back.

In all cases Jack would quickly return to his kind and loving "normal" self once he had vented against those things that had disappointed him. The vacation described at the beginning of this chapter is a good example of hostile behavior resulting from time impatience. You will recall that Jack had set a time in his mind when the family "should" leave for their holiday. While this time was arbitrary and set because

Jack "wanted to avoid traffic," it was not agreed to by Pamela and was a completely unrealistic expectation.

Unrealistic expectations are a major way that people set themselves up for constant, stress-building disappointment and stress itself. When we set goals that can't be met, it's no wonder we end up feeling bitter and hostile toward a world that seems uncooperative, unyielding, and unreasonable. Unrealistic expectations are one type of unhelpful, distorted cognition—and a big one. In contrast, realistic expectations are determined by how others have behaved in the past and by how events and situations have turned out. When we base our expectations on this factual history, we're much less likely to be disappointed and therefore much less likely to pile stress on ourselves. Unrealistic expectations are based instead on our ideals; in our own minds this is how others, events, and situations "should" act, not how they necessarily have acted up until now. The wisest among us hope for the best but don't expect it—and therefore don't hold it against anyone or anything that can't make that steep grade.

Living with a partner's unrealistic and arbitrary standards can be a major strain. Pamela began resenting Jack, cringing in anticipation of his outbursts and resenting herself for not being more assertive with him. Rita often embarrassed Jocelyn with her "diatribes" at wait staff, cab drivers, and almost anyone who disappointed her. And she was disappointed often! Jocelyn tried hard to appease Rita but was often rebuffed no matter how hard she tried. She began feeling that she either had to leave or resign herself to her partner's unremitting intensity and demands.

- *"I never know when she'll be stressed out, irritable, and impossible to talk with."* Jocelyn thought she could never predict when Rita would come home from work feeling peaceful and settled or intense and hostile. She compared Rita to Jekyll and Hyde, a literary analogy I've heard used all too often to describe angry partners. This unpredictability fuels a loss of control and feelings of apprehension on the part of the partner, who is waiting to see which side of his or her loved one will be present at a party with friends; on a vacation, which naturally includes lots of stresses and adjustments (such as when the train leaves late or the hotel has "messed up" the reservation in some way); or at a child's birthday party, where you can usually expect—from factual history!—lots of unruly behavior and noise.

When you can't predict when your partner may react in a way that is scary, embarrassing, or outrageous, you must remain on constant alert. Psychologists call this anxious state *hypervigilance*, which means you can't let down your guard and relax. You must be watchful and prepared for whatever threatening thing may come next. If you can relate to being vigilant for your partner's next outburst, you already know how mentally and even physically exhausting this can be. When you are apprehensive and watchful, your brain and nervous system fuel fight-or-flight symptoms like tight muscles, stomach upset, and increased blood pressure and heart rate, which can impact the quality of your life and even your long-term health. What to do to prevent another anger episode? How do you bring more personal control to the situation to avoid any possibility of another hostile flare-up? You begin to avoid.

- *"I avoid all vacations and travel with Bill as much as possible. This way I know I won't be humiliated by his behavior."* One way to avoid your partner's hostile episodes is to begin to avoid any and all situations that may set him or her off. That's what Jasmine found herself doing. Even though she loved to get out of the house for a few days, she kept close to home because she believed that Bill couldn't take the stress of change to his routines. She recounted a number of holidays when Bill's lofty expectations about how airports, hotels, and other aspects of travel "should" go were dashed by the realities of travel in this real world of delays, overbooking, and weather that can be neither controlled nor often predicted. Bill's tantrums, stressed-out moodiness, irritability, and impatience with all the things that didn't go as planned had occurred often enough that Jasmine now avoided any chance of another embarrassment. When Bill went out of town, she was always "busy" when he invited her to go with him. The couple had not taken a vacation for years, and that suited Jasmine just fine. "It's just not worth it to look forward so much to getting away and then have to deal with Mr. Impatience mumbling, tense, and out of sorts when things don't go his way. I begin feeling so nervous I just dread the next 'disappointment' when a plane is late or we have to look at six hotel rooms before he finds one he likes. I've had it, but feel there is no way to get him to change, so I avoid all events that might be aggravating for him."

- *"I hate doing projects with her. Something is bound to go wrong, and she'll lose it."* How does your partner tend to handle setbacks, problems, and obstacles that arise in completing a task, whether it's cooking a meal together, painting a room, or repairing a leaking faucet? Rita seemed to enjoy challenging herself to learn new skills like a new software program, taking skiing lessons, or trying to fix the computer or a household appliance herself, with no outside help. She seemed to revel in accomplishments of all sorts—except when something went wrong. Jocelyn recalled Rita spending an entire morning trying to retrieve a file that somehow was erased from her laptop. As no resolution seemed imminent, Rita persisted, and a high level of intense mumbling soon turned into loud and explosive cursing and statements of despair as the computer refused to respond the way Rita wished. This was a typical scenario for Jocelyn, who became tenser and inwardly frustrated with these toxic outbursts and the accompanying stress engendered by Rita's unrealistic expectations that she could fix anything and solve any problem if she just tried long enough and hard enough. Well, what was tried was Jocelyn's patience!

Bill just as easily blamed himself, Jasmine, or the kids for "incompetence," "inefficiency," and "procrastination" or "lateness" as he blamed others, situations beyond his control, and any machine that did not live up to his "work-right-every-time" standards. His impatience and hostility were felt by all around him when his unrealistic and lofty expectations were not met. Jasmine dreaded these outbursts and would try to shield the children from Bill's intensity by scheduling them to play outside or be with friends whenever a situation arose that seemed likely to provoke his anger. That covered a lot of ground considering that a blowup could be provoked by any situation where Bill depended on others for a service or task completion!

- *"How can I complain? She just can't help it."* An interesting effect of the free-floating nature of hostility is that you may find yourself starting to make excuses for your partner because hostility just seems to be part of the way he or she is. "Rita is under amazing stress, and she is the major breadwinner," says Jocelyn. "How can I complain too much when her anger is just a by-product of her job? She can't help it—it's just her way." Similarly, Jasmine often excused Bill's intense outbursts as a trait: "just the way he is and probably always has been." She dreaded his intensity and sudden hostile episodes, but felt that she had to accept them if she was to continue to have Bill as her husband. Chapter 10 reviews these and other excuses we make for our partners that can roadblock making the changes we need to.

GETTING OUT OF THE STORM: CHALLENGES AND SOLUTIONS

The dilemma of living with someone you love and want to spend your life with who also acts angry in ways you cannot stand is resolved only by change. Either a Jack suddenly realizes that his hostility and intensity is a serious problem he must address or a Pamela has to learn more life-enhancing and self-protective ways of reacting. Pamela had tried numerous times to get Jack to see his problem and to go into counseling, but he had refused for a long time before agreeing to come see me with Pamela. This book is not for the Jacks of the world but for the Pamelas. For Jack, I wrote *Taking Charge of Anger* (see Suggested Resources), which offers anger management strategies. You may want to recommend it to your partner if he or she seems open to the possibility of learning about anger and taking steps to control it. Here you'll find lots of ideas for what you can do now and the next time your partner's hostility erupts to pollute your life. Of course this is the premise of this book: You don't want to leave the relationship if at all possible, but what now?

What you do now is to put the A–E model from Part I into action. As you read this and subsequent chapters on how to apply what you've learned so far, try to think of ways that you can apply each of these ideas to your own journey with a partner's anger. In the following pages we'll look closely at how Pamela did it.

When I first met Pamela, she seemed depressed and resigned to Jack's actions. I immediately asked her to keep a Daily Log (as described in Chapter 2; a blank form is in the Appendix) of situations where Jack's hostility impacted her mood and emotions. I asked her to record what she thought, felt, and did in response to his anger outbursts. I always like to obtain a word portrait of what is going on, but this log is not just a tool for a therapist to use. I've found that when people have a written record of their own responses—exactly what feelings, thoughts, and actions they took in response to their partner's anger—these reactions end up cemented in the mind in a way that makes them easier to spot when they arise again in the future.

Pamela kept a log over several weeks, and in it she described numerous examples and reiterations of Jack's verbal contempt for anything that didn't go as he expected it to:

• *Other people.* Anyone Jack decided was incompetent set him off, including the baby-sitter who left crumbs on the counter after making herself a sandwich, the cabdriver who took a route Jack thought was "stupid," and a coworker who didn't follow Jack's advice to get his report in a full day early to make their group look good.

• *Objects.* Putting together his son's bicycle soon devolved into Jack throwing a wrench and loudly cursing at the manufacturer, his tools, and the "incompetent" bike designer—whoever he was. Most machines, in fact, were on Jack's list: "As soon as I have to get to a meeting on time, the '%&#!' car won't start. Why does this always happen to me!?"

• *Situations.* Traffic was a bugaboo of Jack's almost every day, thanks to the "lousy," "rude," and "incompetent" drivers. Even the weather was blameworthy: "Damn it! Why do I always get delayed? I can't take another thunderstorm!"

Through this informal log, a picture of how Jack's hostile anger was ruling the family's lives started to emerge for Pamela. Of course Jack's audience was often Pamela or their children since Jack wasn't aiming aggressive anger directly at people he had targeted. This spared Jack from descending into violent behavior that could have been extremely harmful to him as well as to others, but that didn't make the situation much easier for Pamela and the kids, who would invariably become anxious and feel somehow responsible for Jack's tirades. Pamela would often try to comfort Jack or help him see that they could solve the problem if only he "could be patient," for example. As is often the case with children who are exposed to anger outbursts, Pamela and Jack's children felt they had to be especially "good" to please their father and avoid any further scary outbursts. In sum, the whole family was held hostage by the specter of Jack's hostility at home, in the car, or on a trip. Pamela felt she could not predict when he would erupt in anger and was on guard to protect the children from his rough and inappropriate words

> Hostile anger imposes a huge burden on families because they are the ones who witness the outbursts and hear all the venomous criticisms and complaints.

and actions. She felt she had few alternatives but to put up with the small but increasing amount of time that Jack was intense and hostile so she could enjoy the rest of their life together when he was "sweet and fun." The problem was that this smaller amount of time was becoming increasingly harder to endure. With few apparent options, she decided to get help.

Similarly, Jocelyn and Jasmine found that they were expending vast amounts of time and emotional energy feeling apprehensive about their partners' next intense outburst and trying to adjust their lives and schedules to try to keep things calm and peaceful—often without success. Jocelyn's Daily Log revealed that she had begun dreading any changes or adaptations the couple would experience, like repainting their home, going on vacation, or having family stay with them for extended periods. She knew that Rita was likely to "go off" when exposed to even the slightest change from normal routines. Activities that should have been fun now seemed like a burden as Jocelyn anticipated the blowup that seemed to loom in her immediate future. She had not been aware of the toll that Rita's hostility was taking on her optimism and happiness before looking over her log.

Once I had a good idea of Pamela's view of the situation from her statements and her review of her Daily Log, I asked to meet with Jack, who reluctantly agreed to come in. Jack had refused to attend any kind of couple/marital counseling and generally was skeptical about counseling. "We should be able to handle our own problems," he explained. "Our problem is just that I'm under stress and Pamela can't really understand how hard it is for me from day to day. Sure I get a bit irritated at times. Who wouldn't?" Jack was obviously in denial about the impact of his actions on his wife and kids (and probably the people he worked with).

Clearly this couple could benefit from couple counseling, but that was not an option. This left Pamela with two choices: she could get help, or she could put up with things as they were. Pamela summoned up the courage to face her relationship difficulties and was willing to make changes for herself, even though she thought the main problem was Jack. This was not ideal, but life's challenges often are not resolved smoothly and perfectly.

Assessment/Awareness (A)

After I had met with Pamela and Jack, I asked Pamela to complete the RAP to assess how she was currently responding to Jack's hostility. Because of keeping the Daily Log already described, she was much more aware of situations that seemed to trigger his ire and also of her own emotions, self-talk, and actions in response:

Emotions

- Pamela's primary emotion as a result of Jack's anger was **anxiety** and a **low level of fear**—of the next intense outburst and how it would affect others.

> The most common emotional response to hostility is anxiety—the dread that your partner's hostility will break through the surface and produce yet another explosion.

- She also felt **guilty** when she got angry with Jack for "scaring" the kids with his tirades because "He is the breadwinner. He works so hard, and I should be more understanding that he can't help it when he gets mad. He is under so much stress!"

Thoughts and Self-Talk

- These uncomfortable emotions then fueled her theories of why Jack acted this way. Pamela's self-talk included **rationalizing** and **justifying** his actions, along the lines of "He can't help it. He is under stress!"—the same excuse that Jocelyn made for Rita, attributing Rita's hostility to the pressures of her job.

- The partners of hostile individuals also often tell themselves their partner will never change. This kind of resignation typically takes hold after they have tried over and over to convince their partner to change without success. The inability to get your partner to change combined with the conclusion that "he can't help it" or "it's just the way she is" may make resignation feel like a relief from trying in vain to figure out why hostility keeps holding you prisoner. Naturally, the relief is short-lived because it doesn't prevent the emotional fallout of the next outburst.

Actions

- Feeling anxious and resentful kept Pamela (and also Jocelyn) paralyzed, unable to respond differently as she patiently waited for Jack to realize that he "has a problem."

- In an attempt to prevent further episodes of hostile acting out from Jack, Pamela would accommodate her husband by **editing** her own thoughts before expressing them out loud and also by **rescheduling** and **redirecting** their lives to avoid people and situations that had been shown to be incendiary to Jack. Do you use any of these coping methods? If you're not sure, review Chapter 2.

- As we've already discussed, Pamela, Jocelyn, and Jasmine all avoided certain situations and settings to try to minimize their exposure to their partners' hostility. Jasmine wouldn't go on trips with her husband; Jocelyn avoided doing projects with Rita; Pamela steered the kids away from Jack when the setting seemed ripe for an outburst.

- Pamela inadvertently rewarded Jack's hostility by trying to comfort, calm, and reassure him when she saw his ire rising. In effect she was telling him his lack of self-control was acceptable and she would take responsibility for making him feel more at ease.

Boundaries (B)

As you know, it's easy to start out defining what you find unacceptable and acceptable from your partner in vague, general terms. After all, your fondest wish is for sweeping changes, so why narrow down your goals? As you read in Chapter 3, however, well-defined boundaries are necessary because specific boundaries can be enforced, where vague ones leave loopholes. Pamela started out with boundaries like "treat me with more respect," "be more kind," and "handle stress better." When asked to translate these into clear and behaviorally specific language, she came up with the following boundaries.

- **Unacceptable:** Loud talking or yelling when he is upset, no matter what the reason. Cursing, name-calling, and negative comments about another person's character, qualities, or motives are unacceptable as well. Also, loud sighing, shaking his head in disgust, and using sarcasm to put down another are out of bounds for Pamela.

- **Acceptable:** When things don't go as Jack wants, Pamela expects him to use a calm and moderate voice tone (as he would use with a coworker) to express his feelings and concerns. She also expects him to avoid all cursing, name-calling, and pejorative comments about another person's character and personal qualities or directed at things that dismayed him—other cars, computers that did not work, and so forth. She would ask him to focus instead on talking about his opinions, feelings, and needs as he might talk with a valued friend or his brother, whom he was close to (Pamela knew he respected him and would never devolve into losing his cool or having a temper tantrum with him, no matter how much the two disagreed on an issue). He would be too embarrassed for someone he admired to see him act that way, she thought.

COGNITIONS (C)

Once Pamela had drawn new boundaries for interacting with Jack, she could turn to examining her beliefs (C) about herself, him, and the relationship that emerged and guided her feelings and actions with him. It was most important to bring out these underlying cognitions so that unhelpful ideas and thoughts could be replaced with new thinking to support her new boundaries and objectives. You, like Pamela, can review the Beliefs Checklist as well as the list of cognitive distortions in Chapter 4 to help you identify your own unhelpful thoughts. Then, as Pamela did, you can craft a rational (fact-based) belief for each unhelpful belief you identify, reinforced with new thinking and actions. Here are two among those we identified:

Unhelpful belief: "I am powerless to change the situation I am in."

Unhelpful cognitive distortions that sustain this belief:

- **Self-deprecating:** "I just don't have the courage or verbal skills to stand up for myself with Jack."

- **Minimizing:** "If I just let it blow over, he will get more relaxed and things won't get out of control."

Unhelpful actions:

- **Not saying anything:** letting his loud and obnoxious actions slide and trying to change the subject or placate him somehow.

Rational counterbelief: "I control how I feel by changing how I think and how I choose to act."

Rational self-talk (to rebut cognitive distortions):

- "I can and will stand up to him when his anger pushes beyond my boundaries. I have handled harder situations, like when Dad was sick and came through with flying colors!"

- "His hostility cannot be tolerated anymore. It will not just blow over even if I wish it would. I must stand up for what I expect from him."

Rational actions:

- To communicate my new boundaries to him whenever he crosses over the line (as explained below).

Unhelpful belief: "He is much stronger than me and will overwhelm me if I speak up."

Pamela would continue to avoid asserting her boundaries as long as she believed her husband would "overwhelm" her. It is worth noting that Jack had never "overwhelmed" her physically and she did not fear him in that way—but did fear his intense, loud remarks and actions. This belief had to be challenged for her to make progress.

Unhelpful cognitive distortions that sustain this belief:

- **Catastrophizing:** "If I give him a hard time, he will just stay at work longer and come up with excuses to be gone. Our relationship will get much worse."
- **Tunnel vision:** "He is so great with the kids. He is a wonderful dad, and I don't want to do anything to disrupt that."

Unhelpful actions:

- **Avoiding speaking up:** Letting Jack "blow off steam" by removing herself and the kids from the situation. Avoiding as many stressful situations (e.g., shopping with the kids, going out to a busy restaurant) as possible.

Rational counterbelief: "I am a strong and smart person. I have a right to stand up for what I need from Jack and anyone else without fear."

Rational self-talk:

- "If he doesn't like what I say, that's his problem. I am only standing up for myself—what I will tolerate and not. If he decides to stay away, he loses out on being with me and the kids."

- "The fact that he's a great dad doesn't give him the right to yell and disrupt the calm of our family with his anger. If he is less intense, that will help the kids."

<u>Rational actions:</u>

- To assertively communicate her boundaries to Jack and to reinforce them with her actions as discussed below.

Pamela wrote out each of her rational counterbeliefs and supporting self-talk and actions on a separate 3" × 5" card and kept them handy to review at least once a day. These new thoughts and actions began to replace her unhelpful behavior of old the more she rehearsed them in her mind and practiced them directly with Jack.

DENIAL OF REWARDS (D) AND EFFECTIVE EXPRESSION (E)

Up until now it had been hard for Pamela to muster the courage to confront Jack when his hostility had turned up the tension dial to a point where all she wanted was for him to calm down and be quiet. To feel motivated, she needed to see how her current actions could be unwittingly encouraging (rewarding) Jack for his hostile behavior, as discussed in Chapter 5. After reviewing her RAP and her Daily Log as well as her recollections of her ways of coping with Jack over the past few years, she decided she needed to alter the following current behaviors that were providing Jack with a positive outcome.

Current Behavior: Loud and Caustic Voice

When Jack would raise his voice, Pamela would usually stop talking and let him vent his frustrations and anger until he "got it out." Pamela realized that by standing there and listening without setting a boundary she was allowing Jack to use her or others he yelled about as a kind of whipping boy for his ire. Jack got to make himself feel better by displacing his inappropriate anger onto his wife, their kids, and others. He felt better, he often said, when he could "get out his anger." Unfortunately, his emotional venting did not have the same effect on

Pamela and the children, who felt anxious, tense, and often treated unfairly by Jack's intense expressions. Another reward was Jack getting out of situations that Pamela felt he should participate in because either he refused to go or she avoided having him come along due to his unpredictability.

New Assertive Response

Pamela resolved to use assertive "I" statements and actions that were very direct, behaviorally specific, and firm:

• If Jack sat and used a calm tone, she would let him know that she appreciated it.

• When Jack began to raise his voice, Pamela would immediately raise her palm in a "STOP" gesture while saying "Jack, raising your voice is not acceptable if you want to discuss this with me. Let's sit down [to immediately reduce his and her tension] and talk about this calmly."

• If Jack continued to raise his voice, she would not use labels ("You're acting like a maniac/abuser"), she would not mind-read or pathologize him ("Clearly you don't care about me or my feelings!" or "You have a real problem with your anger!"), or in any other way provoke or threaten him. She would just stick to her message with a calm voice, looking directly at him using the "defusing" and nonverbal assertive tools found in Chapter 5: (e.g., the Broken Record: "Jack, I am again asking you to please lower your voice. I will talk calmly with you and expect the same.")

• If Jack still persisted in loud, intense talking, she would call a "STOP," stating: "This feels too intense for me right now. I am stopping and will talk with you later when we can talk calmly." Pamela would get up and leave the situation, ignoring anything further Jack might say as a parting shot, such as "Come back here and talk" or "Why do you always have to put me off!"

Pamela has now communicated with her words and actions that the key to opening the door of communication with her is to use a calm, respectful tone of voice. She would no longer remain present if her husband violated her boundaries.

Current Behavior: Insulting Language

Often Jack would begin cursing or creating insulting names for others as he intensely expressed his displeasure with other drivers, salespersons, waiters, or desk clerks who did not meet his expectations. His actions would occur when they were outside the home and Pamela felt "trapped" into putting up with them and feared embarrassment. He would say these things loud enough that the other might overhear him. In the car he would lose it to an extent that Pamela often worried about her safety or the possibility that another driver would retaliate in a dangerous way. What should Pamela do when trapped in a situation out in public when Jack's behavior went over the top? Again Pamela applied the C, D, and E components of the A–E model.

New Assertive Response

First, she identified her self-talk that was undermining her assertion with Jack. For each unhelpful thought she identified a new way of looking at the situation that would support her new behavior:

• *Old self-talk*: "If I say anything, he will only get worse, and we may have an accident."

• *New self-talk*: "I do not have to listen to this. Yes, he's mad, and I can't make him stop, but I will not look at him or listen to what he is saying. If it begins to feel dangerous, I will ask him [using the repeated "Broken Record"] to safely pull over or to leave the situation. If I'm in a public place, I can just leave the situation and go sit down or sit in the car. I do not have to be a captive of his anger!"

Then, Pamela would ask Jack one time with a calm "I" message to handle the situation differently (e.g., drive more slowly, sit down for a few minutes at the hotel to figure out what to do next rather than yelling at the clerk). As a sample "I" statement, Pamela would look over at him and in a calm voice say: "Jack, I know the traffic is bad and you're upset, but when I see you yelling at other drivers and driving fast, it makes me worry about our safety. Would you please lower your voice and focus on us getting there safely?" If this did not cause him to act differently, Pamela realized she must loosen her muscles, lean back, and try to slow down her breathing as she decided to remove any reward for Jack's actions. She would not debate him about how bad the traffic was or listen to his explanations that he was just reacting to "moron" drivers—not his fault! She had the option of asking to return home and in all cases to let Jack know she was taking a "STOP." Like the "STOP" first described in Chapter 5 where you calmly leave the situation, an internal STOP is used when you can't physically leave but must stop any and all further interaction to defuse conflict and take a stand. Pamela would tell Jack she was taking a "STOP," "switch off," and go inside, trying to relax as much as she could. This internal STOP is the only alternative when you are stuck in a situation with a partner who continues to act out and you cannot physically leave. She would ignore him, not looking in his direction or talking or responding to him or his questions/comments if his voice was intense/loud. She decided to always carry a paperback, magazine, or iPod in her purse to distract herself when such situations arose when traveling with him. If he spoke to her in a way that was calm and friendly, she would let him know she appreciated it and resume normal conversation. If not, she would continue to ignore his words and actions, separating from him quickly when they arrived at their destination.

YOUR OWN JOURNEY WITH A HOSTILE PARTNER

Living with a partner who unexpectedly devolves into a loud, demanding, negative, insulting Mr. Hyde version of the person you know and love is no doubt exacting a huge toll on the quality of your life and relationship. Whatever the reason for the breakdowns into hostility—stress, depression, having had loud obnoxious parents, or the great unknown—this behavior is unacceptable. Sometimes your partner's anger issues are exacerbated by health problems, both medical and physiological/emotional. When is a referral for professional help advisable? Many chronic medical or psychological problems can promote the faces of anger discussed in this book. In particular, the following health issues should be carefully considered as possible contributors to anger and conflict that would require professional referral.

Medical issues

Chronic pain problems (e.g., low back pain, fibromyalgia, myofascial pain syndrome)

Migraine or muscle contraction headaches

Gastrointestinal problems that cause pain and discomfort

Thyroid and other hormone deficiencies

Chronic sleep disturbance (e.g., sleep apnea)

Physiological/psychological problems

Anger/impulse control problems

Alcohol and/or drug abuse or dependency

Major depression

Bipolar disorder

Anxiety disorders (e.g., generalized anxiety disorder, panic disorder)

Attention-deficit/hyperactivity disorder (ADHD)

Any significant psychological disorder that affects mood and emotions

Personality traits/disorder involving narcissism, borderline, antisocial styles

As with Pamela, Jasmine, and Jocelyn, you are clear that you will no longer tolerate unacceptable anger expression, no matter what its

---

Encouraging Your Partner to Get Help

If your partner needs medical or psychological help with one or more of the problems listed or you believe that a problem exists, your assertive approach is likely to set the stage for seeking assistance. The Suggested Resources section of the book offers readings and websites to help you and your partner determine when depression, sleep deprivation, alcohol/drug, or other problems may be contributing to anger problems. I have found that asking a reluctant partner to seek *medical* assistance (e.g., "to manage stress," to evaluate sleep and exhaustion) is a good way to open the door to needed help.

root cause or what explanation is offered. Pamela suggested that Jack have a "nonthreatening" physical exam with his internist since he was complaining so often of stress and tension and would only agree to see a "medical" doctor. As a result, he was prescribed an antidepressant to help manage his mood and emotions and was encouraged to seek stress and anger management counseling, which he subsequently did. Once Jack found Pamela unrelenting in asserting her new boundaries, he was more motivated to seek help in coping with his anger, but he did not change overnight. He reported to her that he was trying hard to be calm when his high expectations were not met and made some progress in derailing his ire at times. However, he definitely needed some continuing professional help in better understanding himself and how to regulate his intense emotions early on, before his anger got the best of him. Pamela's new approach to him created some motivation and momentum for him to deal with his problems, which he did, albeit reluctantly.

Pamela felt better about herself and more calm and in control, even when Jack lost it and she had to assert a "STOP" and leave the situation. She recognized that things wouldn't change right away and that his actions were his responsibility. But she could now separate herself from a life revolving around his episodic losses of control. While she was indeed powerless over Jack, her personal new choices changed the interaction between them from Pamela living her life to adjust to Jack's moods (from happy to angry) to Pamela enjoying the good times with her husband and not participating in his relapses into a meltdown ("I am so sorry. I just seem to lose it even when I am trying so hard to stay cool!").

Pamela's story shows that her life was more peaceful and rich when she gave up trying to manage her husband's anger by constantly "having to" adjust her own actions. A bit like our forefathers, Pamela (and also Jocelyn and Jasmine) declared in words and congruent actions a kind of "declaration of independence" from anxiety, fear, guilt, and disillusionment. My clients who are successful stay the course, understanding that their partners often don't appreciate or easily adjust to this new assertion of boundaries. It's not unusual to have to endure a period of unrest and sometimes increased anger when your partner's old anger patterns fail to reap the old rewards, but most of my clients find it is more than worth it! Staying the course is sometimes hard, but giving in and returning to your old habits of reacting and rewarding your partner's anger will only set you back days and weeks in your journey toward inner, and perhaps, outer peace within your life. Chapter 10 reviews and helps you overcome the many possible obstacles your partner may throw your way and offers help in reversing a possible setback as you force your partner to confront your changes.

In the next chapter you'll learn how you might confront external and intense anger that takes a more malignant twist: aggression.

7

WHEN WORDS *DO* HURT

Rejecting Sarcasm and Verbal Abuse

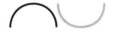

If your partner's anger often comes out as hostility, you know that free-flowing venom is toxic to live with, even when you're not the intended target. Unfortunately, people who express anger inappropriately often have more than one "face" of anger. Sometimes you may find that your partner's anger does seem directed at you personally. At those times it might feel as if your partner has decided to be mean or antagonistic specifically to make you feel uncomfortable or hurt. Naturally this behavior is confusing, coming as it does from someone who supposedly loves and cares for you; of course it shakes your sense of security.

> When words and actions are intended to cause discomfort or harm, whether emotional or physical, they are clearly aggressive and must be addressed for the relationship to survive and thrive.

Make no mistake about it: whether or not violence is involved, aggression can have a toxic impact on your self-esteem, confidence, sense of security, and even health. Therefore it's important to recognize the warning signs of a relationship that is moving in the direction of aggression. Chapter 8 addresses the slippery slope that leads to physical abuse, a form of aggression that is unwelcome in any form, is threatening or even dangerous, and requires professional and/or legal help. This chapter discusses verbal forms of aggression, which, as you'll read later, under "Boundaries," can also be abusive and can ultimately lead to physical aggression.

THE IMPACT OF VERBAL AGGRESSION

Everyone reacts in unique ways to stressful circumstances, but the following signposts are common indicators that your partner has crossed the line into verbal aggression and may be impacting your life in a way that amounts to abuse. Check off any of the following with which you can identify.

❑ You often feel that your expressed feelings and needs are minimized or discounted completely.

❑ Sometimes you feel embarrassed or insulted by how your partner treats you, particularly around others. You sometimes dread going places with him or her for fear of being put down again.

❑ You have been called hurtful names when your partner is mad and don't know how to stop it from happening again.

❑ You can't stand yelling and intense discussion. It feels like you are being criticized and are the focus of your partner's anger way too often.

❑ You feel anxious or fearful of your partner's anger and often find ways of minimizing stress or changing things to avoid his or her anger. You just want to keep the peace.

❑ You often feel insecure and off balance, questioning your partner's love and respect for you. You don't know where you stand.

"Wouldn't I know if I were being abused?" you might ask. Not necessarily. Verbal aggression can be a sneaky form of attack masked as "joking" or "teasing." Even name-calling might seem relatively innocuous when rationalized as the way the person talks to everyone. Because verbal communication is always subject to interpretation, a person who expresses anger through verbal aggression can often elude responsibility

---

**Common Emotional Reactions
to Verbal Aggression**

Do you often feel:

Hurt?

Diminished?

Unrecognized?

Ignored?

Made fun of?

Discounted?

Closed off?

---

by claiming benign intentions. On top of that, *abuse* is a loaded word: many of us don't like to think of ourselves as victimized and don't like to think of our spouses and partners as bullies. This is why interpersonal communications specialist Patricia Evans, who has written extensively about the effect of verbal aggression that becomes abusive, says that identifying your partner's verbal abuse depends on your being able to "recognize and validate" your own emotional reactions.

The tools you gained by learning the A–E model will help you affirm that a joke that doesn't seem funny usually isn't ... that you don't need to resign yourself to the sting of name-calling ... that when someone repeatedly speaks to you and about you in a way that makes you feel demeaned, degraded, and disrespected, you *are* suffering verbal abuse and don't have to.

THE DIFFERENT "VOICES"
OF VERBAL AGGRESSION

Verbal aggression takes several different forms. Which of these do you know and *not* love?

Vince and Melissa are seated at a restaurant with another couple. Vince is animated and enthusiastic about his new position at work. Melissa does not affirm Vince's recent accomplishment in any positive way, but instead throws in sarcastic barbs like "Now Vince gets to play boss and tell a lot of little people what to do. I'm sure he's really looking forward to that!" Vince feels the edge to Melissa's voice but is clearly confused. On the way home she denies she is angry and accuses him of being too sensitive—she was just "joking" with him. With very little effort, Melissa managed to create major discomfort for her husband, leaving him guessing as to what she was really angry about.

> **Sarcasm** is making fun of people or "putting them down" with humor or snide, cutting remarks or via facial expression or tone of voice. The sarcastic person often denies angry feelings, making it difficult to resolve the anger that lies beneath.

Does Your Partner Express Anger as Sarcasm?

At times it may be difficult to discriminate when the line is crossed from humorously joking *with* another person to sarcastically making a joke *of* the other's characteristics or behavior. Some individuals become masters at combining intellectualization and biting sarcasm as a way of letting off the steam of anger through the valve of intellectual riposte and comebacks. Even a slight change in facial expression or a brief comment can feel like a put-down. Imagine you are making a serious point about politics (a tough area in any case), and your partner smiles while saying "Thanks—another example of your brilliant mind at work!!" and then ignores further discussion. How would you feel? Nothing negative has been said, but the intent is suspect, isn't it? Yet when you confront your partner with your negative interpretation, you might be accused of being too sensitive—after all, your partner didn't say anything overtly mean.

One simple way to spot sarcasm is to trust your reaction. No matter what your partner claims to have intended, if it feels like a sarcastic put-down—you feel hurt, embarrassed, demeaned—it probably is. As U.S. Supreme Court justice Potter Stewart once said about pornography, it is difficult to legally define, "but I know it when I see it." If it's an isolated incident that's not characteristic of your partner, there's always a chance that there was no intent to harm, in which case you might want to cut your partner some slack. But if these incidents are frequent, your reaction is probably on the mark, in which case it is important to confront this person with a simple "That felt like a put-down to me. What was your intent in saying that?" While you may get a denial, a pattern of this behavior adds up to a face of anger that must be addressed by a clear boundary that you will enforce.

When you are the recipient of sarcasm, you may feel wounded and belittled yet not know how to interpret what was said or how to respond. Indeed, you can be made to feel that *you* are the problem because you have no sense of humor or you're thin-skinned. In that case, look a little more closely at your emotional reactions to see sarcasm for what it is:

Do you often feel embarrassed by your partner's "humorous" comments about your behavior, appearance, mannerisms, or traits? Melissa would often take the wind out of Vince's sails, putting him down in front of others who mattered to him as a way of acting out her unspoken anger about unresolved issues in their marriage. For fear of further embarrassment, Vince felt he couldn't confront his wife while among their friends, so he would sit there steaming with anger and humiliation.

Sarcasm Cloaked as Humor

"Isn't she the stateswoman! She has an opinion about *everything*!"

"Stuart is really trying to look younger. How do you like the color of his hair? Only his hairdresser knows for sure. Haha!"

"You look great, dear. I didn't know you could fit into that dress. Well, almost!"

"Don't you love the way she can drink all of you under the table? Yes, my wife is quite the drinker!"

The actual words seem neutral or even complimentary, but it is where, how, and when they are spoken that makes them hurtful to the recipient.

Do you frequently feel shaken, confused, or annoyed by your partner's tone of voice, body language, and facial expression that convey disgust, annoyance, or disapproval of you? Similar to sarcasm expressed in words, these actions can be very hurtful. Like sarcasm, your partner may deny he or she meant you any discomfort or harm.

If you feel put down by these kinds of behaviors, you need to place them in the context of how your partner usually treats you and be aware of such actions in the future. Here's an example of another kind of verbal aggression that's important to identify.

Angela wants to repaint the interior of the home she shares with

Nonverbal Communication That May Convey Underlying Anger:

Facial expression:
  Eye rolling
  Head shaking "no" as you talk
  Inappropriate smiling or smirking

Body movements:
  Arms crossed (as if to say "I am not budging!")
  Distractions when you are trying to talk (e.g., fiddling, making noises)
  Leaving the room at a key moment
  Standing to shift focus away from you
  Impatient behaviors (e.g., looking at watch when you are expressing your feelings)

Voice tone and manner:
  Carrying on a loud side conversation
  Speaking to you in a clipped/derisive tone
  Repeating what you said/mocking you
  Interrupting you with casual or joking remarks

her partner, David. She has spent quite a bit of time exploring colors for each room and has brought home paint color samples to show David. He has never really committed to the repainting project and often avoids discussions about it. When she finally asks him to commit himself, they have this discussion:

DAVID: (*Smiles and shakes his head.*) Are we going to have to talk about your foolish ideas for redoing our house again?

ANGELA: David, it's not foolish! This house hasn't been repainted for years. Would you please go with me to the living room so I can show you what I've learned about color and how we can brighten this room?

DAVID: You're obviously unable to listen to anyone but yourself.

You know I don't want to spend the money right now. Don't you have any common sense? Can't you see that you are just wasting your time on this?

ANGELA: Please just consider it. It really is pretty inexpensive if I do the painting myself.

DAVID: *(smug, mocking voice)* Right! You can't even keep the house straightened up. You will just start this and give up like you always do. You can't follow through on anything.

ANGELA: That's not fair—

DAVID: *(Interrupts by repeating Angela's words in a mocking tone.)* That's not fair— *(Continues mocking tone.)* Who brings in the most money in this relationship? I do. You can't even get a decent job. When you do, you can pay for painting yourself. Until then, don't bug me and ask to spend money. Period!

> **Contempt** is criticizing or demeaning a partner's beliefs, traits, mannerisms, appearance, or other permanent or fundamental qualities. Contempt may be expressed without resort to negative labels or obviously abusive language.

Does Your Partner Express Anger through Contempt?

Contempt is a face of verbal aggression that is less subtle than sarcasm but no less insidious. A person can communicate criticism or derogation of your most personal traits, appearance, ideas, or character without cursing or calling you a name but still undermine your sense of self-esteem and confidence. Look at the caustic and critical statements David makes to Angela about her worth, skill, and character. He puts down her effort to beautify their home, treating her with disdain. He undermines her ability to do the job and even shows contempt for her organization and housekeeping abilities. He questions her judgment in pursuing her goal of repainting the house. He also shows contempt for her financial contribution to the relationship, implying that she doesn't have a say until she makes more money.

What David does not do is clearly focus on his partner's proposal and try to listen to Angela and then figure out together whether they can afford to do this project now or when they can afford it. Rather than calmly discussing his feelings and opinions, he makes disparaging remarks about Angela's worth, judgment, contribution, and ability, taking the conversation to a new, personal attack level. So does Juan when he complains to his wife, Maria, that she has thoughtlessly ignored his father's health restrictions in preparing a holiday meal:

> "I can't believe how poorly you listen to anyone. You seem not to care about my dad's health, or you would have realized he can't eat that kind of food. What's the matter with you, Maria? I can't depend on you to use your common sense anymore!"

After enough attacks on her intelligence, abilities, judgment, and character from Juan, what will happen to Maria's confidence and sense of self-worth as a spouse, woman, and worthwhile human being? After enough of the kind of aggression David aims at her, what will Angela likely do to avoid her husband's demeaning criticisms? Maria may begin to question and criticize herself if she internalizes her husband's contempt and starts to believe the negative messages he keeps sending. Angela might avoid having her own ideas, do things behind her husband's back rather than stand up for herself, and begin to resent him and pull away from the relationship. None of these options is a true solution for either woman.

Juan could have expressed his disappointment in a different way, of course, using the "I" messages you learned about in Chapter 5:

> "Maria, I know you spent a lot of time preparing dinner for my parents, and I really appreciated your great effort. My dad suffers from awful gastric reflux and cannot eat spicy food. When he tried to tell you his problem, you didn't seem to get it and repeatedly offered him more food, which of course he couldn't eat. I felt disappointed that you didn't register his problem and was concerned for my dad. Next time I would appreciate it if you would avoid anything spicy or 'hot.' What do you think?"

Notice the focus is on Maria's *behavior*, not on her worth and abilities as a person. Using an "I" message that focuses on his own feelings, opinions, and needs rather than putting down his wife makes Juan's wife more likely to listen and appreciate his feedback. Maria can't force her husband to change his verbal act, but she can certainly make plain when she sets new boundaries that this is how she deserves and expects Juan to talk to her.

**Common Phrases
That Express Contempt:**

"Why can't you—"

"You never—"

"There you go again—"

"I knew I couldn't count on you to do—"

"Why do I even put up with you/your—"

You're hopeless about—"

"You're unable to—"

"You aren't smart [clever, intelligent] enough to—"

"Why even try?!"

These subtle and not-so-subtle personal disparagements not only degrade self-confidence but may contribute to such stress that health and emotional adjustment suffer. They (along with sarcasm) may not seem to fall quite as squarely into the category of verbal abuse as flagrant name-calling and insults, but I must emphasize that they are in fact just as destructive to self-worth and should be viewed with equal concern as new boundaries are being set. And speaking of name-calling:

Leslie and Al have been arguing more intensely lately about the smallest things. While they have always been passionate about their opinions, Al all too often says hurtful and insulting things to Leslie when he gets really mad at her for disagreeing with him. At times he loudly calls her demeaning names and "goes too far" in putting her down, she feels. When we first met, I asked them to try to reach a consensus on a current problem—where they would go for Thanksgiving dinner—so I could observe how they communicated. This is a slice of what I heard:

LESLIE: So, what do you think, Al? Should we go to your mother's or to Florida to see my dad?

AL: I think we should see my mom—she is alone and has been through a lot this year.

LESLIE: That's true, but we haven't seen Dad in two years, and he really wants us to come. I think it's only fair we go since we see your mom all the time.

AL: (*raising his voice and leaning forward*) That's really *lame*. How can you be so *selfish* when my mother does so much for us? She watches the kids and cleans for us all the time because you are so *sloppy* the place looks like a *slum*. Your dad hasn't even come up here to see us in years.

Leslie: (*clearly upset and raising her voice*) "I am *not* a sloppy person. You are the *slob* and *totally insensitive* to the fact I work all day and take care of the kids all night, and you don't appreciate me at all.

AL: There you go. *Whining and moaning.* You can't stand the truth. You're just too *incompetent* to even see how *lousy* you are as a housekeeper.

LESLIE: All you do is put me down. You're a *poor excuse* for a husband and too *self-absorbed* to be a good father most of the time. You don't appreciate me at all. Why bother! I'm out of here! (*Ends the discussion by leaving in tears and does not talk to Al for the rest of the day.*)

> **Negative labeling** is a form of contempt that uses insulting names or disparaging descriptions to demean a partner's personal qualities or behaviors. It is not subtle, but clearly abusive in tone and language.

Does Your Partner Use Negative Labeling to Express Anger?

Listening to their conversation, I wondered how Leslie and Al ever solved a problem. Notice the words in italic that negatively label the other's qualities as a partner, parent, and person. As you read this dialogue, could you sense the level of threat and pain such remarks could create? "Sticks and stones may break my bones, but names *do* hurt"—and they're hard to take back.

Notice that at first Leslie approaches Al with a clear statement of her ideas. When he becomes aggressive by calling her names and insulting her as a partner, she becomes verbally aggressive herself, seemingly as a tactic to defend herself, in a way that "fights fire with fire." While somewhat understandable and often used by my clients to defend themselves, this "stairstepping" of intensity—such as incrementally increasing the volume—only leads to further escalation of conflict that does not solve the original problem, an outcome both Leslie and Al report occurs all too often.

Doesn't Al deserve what he got? He started the verbal abuse, after all, and Leslie only responded in kind. The problem is that Leslie did not clearly identify a boundary for Al's behavior and calmly communicate it until her boundary was heard and considered. By engaging in negative and abusive labeling herself, whether justified or not, she only reinforces a situation in which Al can undermine her with his negative words and subvert resolution of the problem, while also getting her so upset that the conversation ends. Leslie, by getting equally aggressive, gives Al a kind of power to control her emotions if she predictably reacts to his anger this way. He could now justifiably complain that while he "gets a little mad at times and calls Leslie names, *she does it too!*" (a defense that is often used in relationships).

In fact Leslie and Al's marriage was filled with criticism, expressed contempt, and an incredible degree of defensiveness and even stonewalling. These are the "Four Horsemen" that Dr. John Gottman's seminal research has found most undermine a successful marriage and predict divorce. So responding in kind, meeting aggression with aggression, may feel good and justified at the moment, but in the long run it erodes the kind of civil and loving relationship you seek. The A–E model that you've learned in this book offers a better alternative.

ELIMINATING VERBAL AGGRESSION: DRAWING YOUR LINE IN THE SAND

If you've identified with the people depicted so far in this chapter, you have no doubt already asked for relief or tried various ways of getting your partner to stop the verbal abuse. Don't feel discouraged because it seems you've "tried everything" without being able to get your partner to change. Though achieving that would be wonderful, you already know that's not the goal of this book. Success is defined as taking steps to remove yourself from the toxic and wearing din of verbal aggression so that you can shine in ways that fulfill your own dreams and desires. Let's begin by examining the impact of your partner's verbal aggression on you: how you've felt and what you've tried up until now as you get ready to set new boundaries for your partner in the future.

Assessment/Awareness (A)

Once Leslie, Vince, and Angela had completed the RAP and kept a Daily Log of how they thought and felt when verbal aggression occurred, they began to recognize their reactions early in episodes of sarcasm, contempt, and name-calling. This awareness is important because it can keep you from getting so overwhelmed by your own feelings of anxiety, anger, guilt, or fear that you cannot think and respond rationally. Maybe you've found yourself in the same position as Leslie, Vince, and Angela when engulfed by reactive emotions.

Reacting with Anger

Anger was Leslie's predominant emotional reaction to her husband's verbal aggression. Sometimes, she said, she would be so angry and hurt by Al's name-calling that she found herself paralyzed with rage. Yelling back at him or leaving seemed like all she could do. And the more intensely emotional she got, the harder it was to stop and think about what she could say and do to end the conversation. If you've ever been blinded by rage in this way, you know how out of control it can make you feel.

As your level of emotional arousal, also called the "fight-or-flight" response, increases, you are less able to manage what you say and do next. High arousal is often associated with intense acting out of anger and violence. Lack of sleep, stress, not eating well, alcohol and drugs, or being sick or in pain can dramatically increase arousal and set the stage for intense, inefficient, or hurtful acting out of anger.

When she reviewed her RAP responses, Leslie realized she often ended up drawn into the kind of verbal counteraggression you saw in the dialogue you read earlier. When Leslie's anger reached a pain threshold for her, she felt she had to "get away from Al or hit him." She would end up not talking to him for hours or even days at a time (a form of cold anger) to punish him for his abusive behavior. Needless to say, her angry responses were adding fuel to the fire of conflict between them, but she couldn't come up with another way to protect herself. Her friends and family often urged Leslie to leave Al. Caught between not wanting to start over with someone else in her mid-forties and finding the present situation intolerable, she started to realize the only thing she had the power to change was her own reactions to her husband's unacceptable aggression.

Reacting with Fear and Hostility

Vince found himself **fearful** and then **hostile** when Melissa made a sarcastic remark, particularly when she did it in front of friends and his parents. Confused about how to get her to stop, he thought he could only sit there and put up with her nasty barbs, his fear of what she would say next building. He often begged her to respect his privacy before they went out. Since her drinking seemed to promote her sarcasm, he now dreaded Melissa ordering a second or third cocktail: What would she say to embarrass him or others next? On the way home he would feel intensely hostile, driving fast or yelling at other drivers but afraid to confront his wife for fear that she would deny her behavior and tell him he was overreacting or call him a "wimp" who couldn't stand any joking around. Vince's sense of having lost control only heightened his fear and apprehension about what Melissa would say next.

Vince's RAP responses revealed that he often edited what he said to avoid giving Melissa any ammunition to hit him with a sarcastic jibe and often tried to reschedule events, like all-day boating trips and wine tastings where she was likely to drink too much and get nasty again. Vince often tried to keep the conversation away from the topic of his family since she did not like his parents much. He was really tired of having to redirect their lives to head off his wife's sarcasm.

Reacting with Anxiety and Guilt

Angela reported that she mostly felt **anxious** and sometimes **guilty** when David was so critical of her. She worried that he might be right that she often fouled things up and felt guilty that she so often displeased him by asking for things, like the investment in remodeling their house. Was she wrong to even bring it up since he worked so hard and complained about money so often? Was she the cause of his obvious unhappiness in their marriage? Angela's self-confidence crumbled in direct proportion to David's repetitions of contempt toward her. In response, she often rationalized his behavior and apologized and tried to make things right to win back his favor.

How Do You React to Your Partner's Verbal Aggression?

- Do you find yourself overwhelmed by your partner's hurtful statements?

- Which of the three—Vince, Angela, or Leslie—do you identify with most?

- How do you find yourself reacting emotionally when your partner is verbally aggressive?

Keeping your own Daily Log and completing the RAP is a great place to begin this exploration. Your motivation to do something about the unpleasant or even emotionally damaging status quo should begin with a careful assessment of the impact of your partner's verbal aggression on your own feelings and daily life.

- How much are you adjusting your thoughts, choices, possibilities, and actions to avoid or cope with your partner's hurtful expressions of anger?

- Is this acceptable?

- Are you ready to define new boundaries for your partner's actions?

If so, start to think of how you would like him or her to treat you in the future.

Boundaries (B)

How much biting sarcasm, how many put-downs, and how much name-calling from your partner do you find acceptable? At what point does your confidence, self-esteem, or sense of self-worth begin to diminish? These are the questions you need to answer to set new boundaries regarding verbal aggression. At the risk of putting words in your mouth, let me be very direct about where I draw the line: **I believe that verbal aggression at any level should be intolerable to both you and your partner.**

Why? Because verbal aggression is often described as a form of abuse that, if unchecked, can lead to disastrous consequences for you, your children, your parents, or other loved ones who live with you. The

National Coalition against Domestic Violence (NCADV) and the Centers for Disease Control and Prevention (CDC) both describe verbal aggression as part of a continuum that can end in "Intimate Partner Violence" if not stopped (see the table below). Both have compiled lists of nonphysical but destructive verbal actions that can contribute to relationship violence and possible injury, either emotional or physical.

Notice how many of these behaviors fall within this chapter's definition of verbal aggression. Keeping in mind the seriousness and potential consequences of hurtful statements, would you permit another adult to verbally abuse or undermine the self-worth of a child you love? Despite the fact that virtually none of us would allow anyone to undermine a child's self-esteem or confidence in this manner in our presence, many of us permit our partners to say similar mean and humiliating things to us and continue to put up with it in the hope that it will change—that somehow our partners will see the light.

The only solution is to agree that **no verbal aggression is acceptable**. This is a clear boundary that I believe should be a foundation of any intimate relationship.

For Angela and Leslie, who decided that their partners' contemptuous remarks were completely unacceptable, the boundary was simple to define: no derogatory, demeaning descriptions, characterizations, putdowns, or negative labels used by their partners, David and Al, would be tolerated any longer. Instead, Leslie and Angela expected their partners to express their ideas, feelings, and needs using a calm and friendly tone

Emotional Abuse (NCADV, 2009)	Verbal Forms of Emotional Abuse (CDC, 2009)
• Putting partner down • Making partner feel bad about herself/himself • Name-calling • Making her/him doubt sanity • Playing mind games • Humiliating partner • Making partner feel guilty	• Humiliating the partner • Withholding information • Doing/saying something to make the partner feel diminished or embarrassed • Harming a partner's sense of self-worth • Name-calling

of voice, free from personal put-downs and negative labels. For example, Leslie wrote defined boundaries for Al that were clear and behaviorally specific:

- **Unacceptable:** Any negative names or labels used to describe or define Leslie's personality or behavior. Al's frequent description of Leslie as "limited," "incompetent," and "useless," often said in anger, would not be tolerated no matter what Al was feeling or why he was upset. Getting "in her face" (closer than three feet) when he was angry would also be out of bounds.

- **Acceptable:** If Al had a problem or complaint about Leslie, he was to describe the specific problematic behavior, his feelings, and what he requested of her instead. She required that he speak to her in a calm and friendly tone, like how he spoke to his clients at work, staying at least three feet away from her. She expected him to find opportunities to praise her when he was pleased by something she did.

Because Melissa's sarcastic statements were a bit harder to define, Vince spent considerable time trying to describe what behavior was unacceptable. He decided that he would describe from Melissa's statements, tone of voice, and manner what felt most insulting and demeaning to him. Even though she often denied she was angry or meant to cause him any discomfort (e.g., "Vince, what are you *talking* about? I was only pulling your leg. Get a life!"), he reviewed his Daily Log and defined these unacceptable behaviors for Melissa:

- **Unacceptable:** Melissa's interrupting his storytelling or conversation with their family or friends once Vince had the floor. Also, Melissa's making light or fun of his accomplishments or actions at work or revealing embarrassing personal information about him or their marriage. He thought about these examples to illustrate his boundary to Melissa if necessary:

> "Vince *never* confronts anyone at work. He just wants to be loved, and he has certainly accomplished that! Too bad he can't get a raise!"

> "I have to work. Vince can't support us on his own, but *I* don't mind [Melissa sighs]; he's a good dad."

> In response to someone else's sexual joke or story: "Of course,

Vince couldn't care less about sex. It's like he would rather watch American Movie Classics since his prostate problem. Oh well!"

• **Acceptable:** To quietly listen to him with full-faced attention when he had the floor, without interrupting. To use a tone of voice that showed interest and concern and to keep all personal information about Vince between the two of them. If Melissa was upset with him, to discuss it in private in a calm and respectful manner.

After considering the boundaries Leslie and Vince crafted for their partners' verbal aggression and employing the ideas offered in Chapter 3, think about your own relationship, perhaps after reviewing your Daily Log. Try to establish one or more boundaries to clearly define how your partner's current behavior is unacceptable to you and the kind of actions you would appreciate in the future.

Cognitions (C)

Unhelpful beliefs and dysfunctional self-talk (Chapter 4) can undermine your ability to stand up for new boundaries. Vince concluded that his anxieties and apprehension about what Melissa might say to embarrass him had roadblocked his efforts to assert himself in the past. He reviewed the "Beliefs Checklist" in Chapter 4 as a guide to identifying beliefs that had immobilized him with fear and anxiety. For each he crafted a fact-based, positive belief that he would reinforce with new self-talk and assertive actions, shown in the table on the next page.

Vince decided to write out each new, helpful belief on a 3" × 5" card and vowed to read it over multiple times each day and whenever he felt anxious about Melissa's mood or anger. We also identified cognitive distortions that seemed to fuel his old beliefs and trigger anxiety. For each we crafted some example rebuttals that he could practice saying to himself in his imagination to set the stage for thinking more clearly when Melissa's anger was aroused. Here are three examples. Keeping in mind Chapter 4, note that each rebuttal focuses on the **facts and/or plans how to achieve an emotional or behavioral goal.**

Rationalizing

"Melissa can't help the way she acts in public. She gets caustic because she's had too much to drink or she is feeling uncomfortable."

Transforming Your Beliefs

Unhelpful Beliefs	New Helpful Beliefs
"I can't handle Melissa's anger."	"I control how I feel by changing how I think and act."
"Her biting remarks overwhelm me."	"I am powerful over myself and choose to change."
"Nothing works to get her to change."	"Melissa may not change, but I can and will."
"She will change if I give it enough time."	"Time does not change things. My new thinking and actions will change things for me. Her changes are up to her."

Rebuttals (to keep in mind and try to use):

"Melissa's actions embarrass me, but there is no good excuse for her to put me down, ever."

"She chooses to overdrink and controls what she says and must experience consequences in my refusal to accept sarcastic remarks any longer."

"I have a perfect right to expect to be treated with respect by my wife, no matter how she feels."

Tunnel Vision

"Most of the time she is very respectful of me. It's only when she's upset that she puts me down."

Rebuttals:

"Sarcasm is unacceptable no matter what other good qualities she has. I will state emphatically it is not acceptable!"

"Even though it seems to occur only when she's mad, it hurts and embarrasses me and is an unacceptable way for her to express her anger. It happens often enough that I need to raise it as an issue with her."

Self-Deprecating

"How can I criticize her when I know she has to put up with my long hours and so much business travel?"

Rebuttals:

"Even if she *is* angry about my being gone a lot, I will encourage her to tell me her feelings directly and not put me down in front of others or humiliate me at home."

"My work hours are invested to provide for our family and not an excuse to say mean things. If she wants me to work less, she should discuss alternatives with me and not put me down."

Regarding the contemptuous expressions of anger that Angela and Leslie were receiving from their partners, a similar approach identified old thinking and new beliefs and rebuttals to support their boundaries. For example, Angela's new beliefs and helpful self-talk, written on cards she kept in her purse for quick reading, included the one shown in the box here.

New Helpful Belief

"I am a valuable and capable person and deserve to be treated respectfully at all times."

Supportive Self-Talk:

"No matter how much stress David is under, I deserve a calm and friendly voice and words."

"My life can and will change, no matter what David decides to do."

"If he is unhappy and leaves me, I will survive and my life will be a lot more peaceful. If he changes and stays, that would be wonderful, but I am okay regardless!"

Leslie's examination of her thinking revealed that her loud and angry reactions to Al's name-calling and contempt were fueled by the belief that "being aggressive is the only way to stop aggression." She had learned this in childhood as she witnessed her parents' almost nightly verbal fights that escalated as each tried to one-up the other by getting louder and saying something more hurtful. A new helpful belief and supporting self-talk were expressed on the card shown below, which she kept handy to read often, reminding her of her new boundaries and goals.

Now Vince, Angela, and Leslie needed to decide how to express their new boundaries and beliefs to their partners in a way that was not provocative, but firm and rich in information as to how the partners were expected to express their anger differently in the future. In all cases, the three focused on not rewarding their partners in any way for their old aggressive statements and voices.

The Art of Verbal Self-Defense: Denying Rewards (D) and Assertive Expression (E)

Now that you are clear about your new boundaries, you must find a time, place, and situation that are conducive to communicating your expectations when your partner is willing, ready, and able to listen and respond. As pointed out in Chapter 5, good timing sets the stage for success in getting your points across. Vince waited until the next morning while the two were having coffee together to confront Melissa with her sarcastic behavior of the previous evening. She was sober, rested, and

---

New Helpful Belief

"I have a right to ask for kind and calm words when Al is upset with me. I can use calm and kind words to assert exactly what I expect from him."

Supportive Self-Talk:

"The fact is that I am bright, capable, and kind and deserve to be spoken to with dignity and respect at all times, no matter how Al is feeling."

"I can best react to Al's anger with calm and firm statements of how I expect to be treated. If I don't like what he says, I can leave or refuse to talk further."

presumably not distracted by others or a party situation. He informed her that he would no longer go to great lengths to edit, redirect, or shift his plans to minimize her possible anger. He would let her know immediately with direct eye contact and a combination statement ("Excuse me?") and corresponding hand gesture (palm raised) to signal her that he was talking and did not want to be interrupted. Upon a further interruption he would immediately use the "Broken Record" strategy of calmly repeating his "STOP" message, looking directly at her with a firm facial expression. The same tactic would be used when she would begin to tell a joke at his expense or begin to relate embarrassing personal information to others. Once she stopped her statement, he would say to her: "Thank you." If others were present, he would then continue the conversation as if nothing was wrong. This tactic incorporated the underlying message that he would no longer sit helplessly by when he felt Melissa was disrespecting him with her cutting remarks. If she failed to respond to his "STOP" statement, he could always excuse himself and leave to underscore the idea that he was no longer tolerating sarcasm. Here is the way he approached it as they had breakfast together at home. Note Vince's use of an "I" statement:

> VINCE: Last night I felt very humiliated and embarrassed when you told our friends about me getting passed over for a promotion *again*. This is very personal information, and I would have told them myself if I had wanted it known. Please check with me before telling anyone anything personal about me that could be embarrassing. When in doubt, please don't tell it. In addition, you've been saying cutting things to me lately, calling it "joking around." Sometimes I find what you say funny, but often it hurts and is unacceptable. From now on I'll tell you immediately to stop any remarks that seem sarcastic and hurtful to me.

> MELISSA: Vince, you are totally too sensitive! No one seemed to care about your job, and you are overreacting as usual. And I am not trying to hurt you. Ever!

> VINCE: I'm not going to discuss my feelings further as they are important to me even if you minimize them. From now on if I feel you are beginning to say something demeaning or sarcastic about me I will signal you to please stop by looking directly at you and raising my palm. I will kindly say "Excuse me?"

and then say something like: "Let's talk about something else, okay?" while shifting the discussion. If you persist, I will repeat what I just said until you stop or I leave the situation. I will try not to embarrass you if we're with others—I might excuse myself to get some water or go to the bathroom—but I will not be embarrassed ever again without speaking up.

MELISSA: You wouldn't really do that, would you?

VINCE: I am very serious. I will no longer tolerate your sarcasm or embarrassing statements about me when we're alone or with others.

Vince has now laid down a clear boundary and informed his wife in advance of how he intends to respond to her sarcastic anger in the future. Rather than get into a discussion about what sarcasm is or whether Vince is "too sensitive" about a given remark, Vince made clear that if *he* felt uncomfortable with it he would ask for a stop. **It's important for the partner who feels put down or injured by the remark to define what is acceptable and what is not.**

Imagine you're at a party and you tell a joke that is slightly off-color, having no intention of making anyone uncomfortable. If someone is offended, do you accuse the person of being too sensitive, or do you apologize and avoid such jokes with that person in the future? You probably recognize that the impact of what you say should guide whether or how you say similar things in the future. Your partner should be informed that you expect him or her to do the same.

Angela and Leslie both decided to communicate new boundaries to their partners that they would not tolerate further contemptuous or abusive statements in any form. Angela found a good time to tell David her new expectations and responses if *she* finds his words objectionable.

ANGELA: David, in the past few months you have often used critical and demeaning descriptions of me to my face or around the kids. For example, you have demeaned my taste and judgment about making our home more presentable, have mocked my ideas many times, and put me down in front of our kids by criticizing how I do things like keep the house clean and presentable. You don't just offer a suggestion, but put me down as a person. Your put-downs make me feel worthless, embarrass me, and hurt unbelievably. I will not tolerate your hurtful words any longer.

DAVID: You are so overreacting! Look at all I do for you and the kids. I'm under stress, and I get angry and say things I don't mean sometimes. Can't you be more understanding?

ANGELA: I will never understand put-downs of me as a wife or person. If I believe in my mind you are saying something mean to me, I'll ask you to stop and raise my palm like this (*raised palm facing David*). If you stop, I'll continue the discussion with no further comment. If you continue with mean put-downs, I'll get up and leave for at least twenty minutes. From now on you can tell me anything you want with calm and kind words. Tell me what you would like to see me do differently or any ideas you have about what we should do as a couple. I will listen and consider what you say. But say it calmly as you would to a coworker or our neighbors or I am off to you.

DAVID: I can't believe you really think I'm so mean and terrible. Wow!

ANGELA: I think you're a good man or I wouldn't stay with you. It's the way you act and what you say to me when you're mad that I cannot tolerate anymore.

PUTTING VERBAL AGGRESSION TO BED: SOME FINAL THOUGHTS

Take any form of verbal aggression seriously. I believe there is no action in a relationship that so quickly degrades and undermines personal and mutual respect. Much research suggests that verbal aggression may be the first step on a slippery slope that pulls you and your partner down in ways that you may not believe possible. Put-downs that seem casual quickly cross a line when both parties are not in total agreement that they're funny and benign. And even then, unless they are rare, they often take on a life of their own and mushroom into a bad habit. An unwelcome side effect is that disparaging others you love or using negative labels in jest may be copied by your partner and other family members and then come back to haunt you. Suddenly you realize that the barbs are no longer funny and no longer innocuous. Don't give them the chance to reach that stage; set a standard for civil, mutually respectful, and kind communication all the time.

No couple plans to have an abusive relationship. None of my angry clients planned to become abusers or act mean to loved ones. But verbal sparring and put-downs yield to threats and actual violence all too often. I hope this does not describe you, but if it does, you'll find help in Chapter 8. If it does not, take steps now to set and reinforce life-enhancing boundaries.

8

THREATS AND BEYOND
Staying Off the Slippery Slope
of Physical Abuse

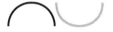

No rational person plans to be physically abusive.

No one plans to be a victim of physical abuse.

Yet you may find yourself in a relationship where verbal aggression and other inappropriate faces of anger have begun to evolve into more serious forms of physical touch.

How has this happened? Why does your partner get so angry? What has brought threats, unwanted physical touch, or even violence into your relationship?

It's beyond the scope of this book to discuss the pathways that lead some people to become violent or to accept a violent partner. Why a partner is violent can be addressed best by a mental health professional who can evaluate the situation in light of the current research into personality development.

Yet you may find yourself so invested in understanding why your partner is this angry that your own needs to feel safe, calm, and secure in a predictable relationship have fallen by the wayside. When was the last time you asked yourself what living with someone who may make you feel physically threatened is costing you emotionally, in self-esteem, and in personal safety?

If your relationship has developed into threats, physical touch, and even violence, it is *past* time to act. Do whatever it takes to ensure your safety and the quality of your life. If you can do so by making changes that preserve your relationship, that may be the best outcome. Reading this book shows that you wish to restore your most important relationship to something that feels calm and loving. Yet sometimes it is essential to separate for your safety and to preserve any possibility of resolving the anger and underlying issues that pull you apart. Or you may have chosen a partner who is incapable of change and you are forced to make separation permanent. These issues are tough to address and require more careful consideration than is often found in the misguided advice that many people in your position receive from well-meaning family, friends, and even some professionals:

"If he touches you, you must immediately end the relationship."

"Abusers *never* change. If you are abused, your only option is to leave."

"You must stick it out no matter what. All couples go through tough times. It will get better."

"I'm sure he/she is just under a lot of stress/pressure. You have to be understanding and try to keep things calm. Just try to avoid him/her when mad."

When you're in the thick of it, it's often hard to see how low levels of aggression, perhaps beginning with verbal slings and angry retorts, can be the beginning point of a journey that no one signed on for and along which someone gets hurt. All relationship violence begins with conflict. At first it may not seem scary at all, and its road signs may be overlooked or explained away as unimportant squabbles or explainable intense exchanges. Even if your partner's aggression is strictly verbal at this time, it's important to learn to read the signposts on the way to violence and understand what you can do to derail the engine that's taking you on this unwanted trip. If you're already heading into this dangerous territory, it's critical that you learn when and how to communicate this firm and unyielding boundary:

Any physical touch in anger is unacceptable, no matter who initiates it, what the rationalization or reason, or how it is expressed, other than self-defense.

NOT ALL AGGRESSION IS THE SAME

Whether aggression can be resolved depends largely on the extent to which your partner understands he or she is wrong and wants to change. Scientists who have studied relationship aggression don't view all aggressive persons as having the same backgrounds or characteristics. Summarizing across this research, aggressive people seem to fall into two basic categories. One type of aggressor can't effectively identify or regulate anger arousal and may also have poor coping skills for expressing anger. If this is your partner, he or she may feel all the standard physiological sensations of increased heart rate, muscle tension, and sensory awareness, but can't seem to derail this cascade of events. Researchers P. H. Neidig and D. H. Friedman have called these individuals "expressively aggressive," meaning that their expression of anger is not well regulated and they need to learn emotional, self-control, and anger management strategies. As shown in the sidebar on the next page, the prognosis for making changes is good when these people seek counseling because they're capable of sincere remorse and typically don't have more severe personality dysfunction.

Quite different in intent and much less amenable to change is the partner who displays *instrumental aggression*, which arises from more deep-seated personality dysfunction. The instrumentally aggressive partner wants to be in control and to intimidate his partner to get what he wants. Aggression is a means to an end, and this person may turn "anger" on and off quickly based on what is called for. In other words, the instrumentally aggressive person uses aggression to intimidate and may not experience high levels of arousal.

It's crucial to know whether your partner exhibits signs of this malignant form of aggression:

• Does your partner use anger to exert power? If so, he or she may not lose control of arousal.

Two Types of Anger Expression

Those who are *expressively aggressive*:

- are often highly emotionally aroused

- express anger because they can't control their arousal

- gradually escalate their inappropriate expressions of anger

- take responsibility for their anger actions and feel and express credible remorse, though the partner often accepts responsibility as well

- have a better prognosis because they are highly motivated to change. Education and therapy can often help them alter the way they express anger by helping them learn emotional regulation and coping skills.

Those who are *instrumentally aggressive*:

- use aggression to control and punish the other person, to achieve an objective that is probably not shared by the victim

- often come from families filled with violence and neglect

- become violent without any clear trigger

- rapidly escalate their expressions of anger

- show no credible remorse

- often have serious personality traits like narcissism, borderline, or antisocial

- play a fixed role of perpetrator to your fixed role of victim

- have a much less positive prognosis since they have little motivation for counseling. They respond best to legal boundaries (e.g., threat of punishment).

• Your partner may apologize or try to atone for violence with gifts or kind acts while still having little internal understanding of the impact of his or her actions and little remorse that eliminates or reduces future aggression. Thus aggressive behavior is repeated again and again, with a cycle of apologies and pleas for forgiveness.

• Again, it's beyond the scope of this book to explain a particular individual's instrumental aggression, but this problem is usually the result of deep personality problems stemming from childhood abuse, neglect, or detachment from parent figures. This makes treatment difficult and behavior change unlikely without a full commitment to therapy. In some cases, change never occurs, and the instrumental aggressor has a series of intense, violent relationships with unfortunate partners who will be hurt repeatedly.

If your partner seems to fit the instrumental aggression profile, seek counseling to help you decide whether this relationship is viable and what your options are. Unless your partner is motivated to seek intense counseling to address underlying personality problems, aggression is highly likely to continue. No matter what your partner does, you must set firm and unyielding boundaries that tolerate no acts of aggression and seek professional counseling for yourself right away.

In my practice I don't work with those who feel no remorse or who hurt others for purely selfish reasons. I enthusiastically offer counseling, however, to those who have the potential for change and who sincerely feel remorse when they say and do aggressive things. In a twist on Rabbi Harold Kushner's book *When Bad Things Happen to Good People*, I view people who fit the expressive aggression profile as fitting the designation "When Good People Do Bad Things." And as you saw in the sidebar, the prognosis is good if your partner is among them and is motivated to change. Your partner may need to seek counseling to learn to better regulate emotions and expression of anger, or couple treatment may be in order if mutual escalation is occurring. Regardless, you will set new boundaries and make changes that improve the quality of your life in this relationship.

STOPS ALONG THE ROAD TO PHYSICAL VIOLENCE

Assuming, then, that your partner's aggression falls into the expressive category, you need to start making good decisions so you can divert your relationship off the path of violence and onto the path of resolution. As aggressive behavior proceeds from less to more intense, moving from intimidation to physical acting out of violence, there are certain kinds of behaviors you can observe that tell you where you are on this unpleasant journey. Where are you and how much farther are you willing to go before drawing a firm line in the sand of this relationship?

Threats

The first signs of potential physical abuse are threats of violence, whether implicit or boldly explicit. The aggressive partner threatens bodily harm. Is this just a ploy? Does he really mean it? It is important to take such threatening statements seriously, as they are abusive in themselves, even if the partner never follows through with the threatened actions. Other than being physically attacked, there is probably no event that elicits immediate fight-or-flight body arousal (in the form of fear) faster than when injury or death seems possible. This is why threats are intolerable at any level. Your most basic needs for safety and security (as discussed in Chapter 3) are undermined by threats, and they must not be permitted to continue.

Threats come in both subtle and overt packages. Have you been threatened in a way similar to any of these nonspecific, yet intimidating, statements?

> "If you don't shut up, I will shut you up!"
>
> "[Glaring and moving closer] You had better do it or you will be very sorry."
>
> "[Shouting] I am *so angry* I'm going to lose it any minute!"
>
> "I will never let you do that—don't push it!"
>
> "[Standing up/towering over the partner] Don't make me do something we will both regret!"

Each of these statements threatens you without ever stating outright what the harmful actions will be: Punching? Slapping? Pushing? Even though what is being threatened remains ambiguous, you immediately get the message: your safety is at risk.

> In contrast are the overt, all-too-clear threats of specific acts of violence:
>
> "I will shut your mouth for you with this" [raises fist].
>
> "You will never get out of this room unless you admit that you caused this whole argument!"
>
> "If you don't shut your mouth, I will" [describes violent act].
>
> "I could kill you, I'm so mad!"

Needless to say, any threat to your person should be taken very seriously, particularly if it describes exactly what your partner intends to do. But you probably don't need to be told this. We are hardwired to react immediately to such threats with the adrenaline-fueled fight-or-flight response. While getting out of the situation and seeking safety is the sensible way to flee or withdraw, many victims of violent threats withdraw by acceding and submitting, behaviors that often only reinforce and encourage bullying/intimidating threat behavior. Many people naturally react to a partner's threats by using all the diversionary tactics discussed in Chapter 2—editing, redirecting, rescheduling, and subjugating their own needs—to avoid any possibility of being hurt. In the process, the relationship can tilt to a dominant–submissive life pattern that ultimately exploits the "weak" partner.

How would *you* respond to such threats? Would you stop asking for your boundaries to be respected? Would you fear loss and pull back from expecting your needs be considered? It's easy to say no, but threats can be very scary and immobilizing, particularly when you've built your life around a partnership that now seems on the verge of collapse.

Gestures That Intimidate without Touching

Hunter and Charlotte often thought of themselves as a loving but intense couple. They were passionate in the way they approached their careers, spending long hours working to make partner in their respective law firms. They both described themselves as intense; hostility was their most common face of anger. Neither of them suffered fools well; both could be counted on to tell off the slow clerk, inefficient airline employee, or waiter who did not measure up to their standards for good service. While Hunter's anger was expressed mostly with a loud voice and biting sarcasm, Charlotte's anger started to go "beyond the pale" all too often. She would sometimes get within inches of Hunter's face and scream at him at the top of her lungs, making it impossible for Hunter to move away from the situation without touching Charlotte, which he did not want to do in anger. Lately she had begun throwing whatever was close at hand at the wall or smashing things, often narrowly missing him. Sometimes she would threaten to damage something that was important to him, like a framed photo of him with his parents or a plaque he had been given for success at work.

Charlotte's behavior was pushing Hunter to greater and greater heights of anger and frustration that he was barely able to contain.

Hunter tried to back off and suggest they separate at such times, which only seemed to inflame the situation. He was afraid of what Charlotte might do and what he might do to her in response. He wanted the intensity to stop but found it hard to derail once an argument had begun.

Do you find yourself feeling intimidated when your partner does things like the following that seem to threaten you with harm yet you are not physically touched?

- Getting so close to you when angry that you feel uncomfortable or intimidated

- Yelling or screaming so loudly in your face that your ears ring

- Standing in your path so you cannot exit the situation or leave the room/house

- Throwing a punch in the air that almost hits you but misses, causing you to flinch or rear back in fear

- Throwing or smashing things, particularly if objects are thrown in your direction

Touching That Escalates the Chance of Violence

Sam and Lacey had three children, a lovely home, and a great life in a wonderful neighborhood. They seemed like the perfect couple to their friends and family. Yet there was a dark side to their relationship that only they knew about and tried to deny to themselves. Over the past year Sam had become increasingly aggressive when the two had a disagreement. He would curse in a loud voice and make disparaging remarks about Lacey as a wife and mother. Lacey tried to cope by avoiding any subject or situation that might set Sam off. Often her editing, redirecting, and apologizing tactics seemed to work as long as Sam was not too stressed and had no more than a few beers.

What was disconcerting were the all too frequent instances when Lacey could not seem to head Sam off from getting so angry that he frightened her. He had begun to call her names and use language to insult her that she never believed she would tolerate from anyone, yet she tried to calm him down or give in to his demands to keep the peace. He would sometimes get in her face and hold her arms so she could not leave to go to their bedroom to let him "chill out." He would stand in front of her, pushing her back with his chest and body so that she sometimes felt that she was held "hostage" until he screamed out everything he wanted to say. Lacey felt demoralized, intimidated, and hopeless that this situation would get better.

Recently Sam had broken into the bathroom where Lacey had locked herself in to get away from his anger. He got in her face and would not let her leave until she "listened" to him. She cried and pleaded with him to let her leave, but he held on to her arms and blocked any movements, which made her feel even more frightened and disconsolate. When she told him how mean and abusive he was, Sam would retort that "I've never hit you! How can you call me an abuser? You're the one who makes me so mad that I do these things." Lacey felt powerless to respond to such defensive statements and had to admit he had never hit her. Also, these episodes "don't occur all the time," she rationalized. Why, then, was she so scared and at the end of her rope? She felt like a failure as a wife, a belief that was constantly confirmed by her husband's contemptuous and mean statements to her.

Clearly Sam's verbal abuse had grown into frequent use of physical tactics to hold, block, or restrain Lacey in ways she found abusive. Using physical force of any kind to attain a goal of getting the other to listen or making the other stay is intolerable at any level, no matter what the partner's intention is (e.g., "I only want to get you to hear me out/to make things better"). Does your partner use any of these, tactics similar to Sam's, to coerce you?

- Holding on to your hands or arms to direct you to do something your partner desires

- Hugging or holding in any way that is unwanted

- Sitting or lying on top of you to restrain your movements

- Blocking you from leaving or directing your movements by pushing, holding, chest blocking, or using any other restraint

Unmistakable Violence: Physical Abuse

Janice wondered how her marriage could have come to this low point. She couldn't believe it, given how much she still loved her husband, Frank, and how good their relationship had once been. Janice had read numerous self-help books on "victims of abuse" and had spoken to her friends and pastor, all of whom told her she should leave Frank and get counseling for herself. But Janice said she still loved him and felt he was a good man who had serious anger problems. Frank had been an attentive husband and good provider who was tender and loving with their three teenaged children, except when he was irritated about something. He had begun to lose his temper more frequently over the past two years, which Janice felt had a lot to do with his losing his former job and having to work for less money and status. Frank had seemed very depressed and moody and was prone to drink alcohol to cope with his "stress" more frequently over this period. His anger would get the best of him with drivers, neighbors, and occasionally her and the children when he felt they were doing something purposely to upset him (e.g., making noise with loud music, failing to get homework done, asking him to help around the house when he was too tired).

When intensely angry, Frank would sometimes lose it and get in Janice's face, screaming that he couldn't take the stress anymore. She often asked him to see his physician or a therapist to get on a medication or get counseling to help him with his anger and mood. Frank refused help ("What do you think I am? Crazy? I'm just under a lot of pressure and I can handle it."), yet continued to subject Janice to his rages. Lately he had begun to block her exit until she stood there and listened as he raged on. When she tried to leave, he would push her back or restrain her from moving. On a number of occasions Janice reported that Frank hit her with his open hand to "get her attention" and had kicked at her when she managed to slip by him to leave. Recently he had pushed her away from him, and she fell backward into a table, injuring her back, which was still sore from the blow. Immediately, Frank was solicitous and apologized repeatedly for his actions, blaming his behavior on being "too stressed" to think clearly. The yelling, threats, physical intimidation, and now the hitting had become too much for Janice to bear. This pattern of physical violence followed by apology and attempts at atonement is all too common among partners who are physically abusive and must be stopped immediately.

Does your partner show any of these behaviors of physical violence? How have you coped so far, and how has it worked for you?

- Pushes you with an open hand or body (e.g., bumps you aside with his hip, pushes you forward when you are walking "too slowly")

- Slaps you with an open hand while protesting that he/she has never hit you with a fist

- Punches you with closed fist

- Throws something at you or hits you with an object

- Pushes you down or trips you

- Touches you in any way that hurts (e.g., pinching, hair pulling, poking with finger)

- Threatens or acts aggressively with any weapon or object that could injure (a knife, fork, bottle, tool, gun, etc.)

- Apologizes and asks for forgiveness ("Will never do it again") yet will not get help for his/her anger

WHERE ARE YOU ON THE SLIPPERY SLOPE?

In Chapters 6–8 you've read about what is essentially a continuum of overt inappropriate faces of anger, from hostility all the way through physical violence. You could view you and your partner as climbing (reluctantly, at least on your part) a ladder that could ultimately end in life-threatening abuse. Much research shows that physical violence often begins with contemptuous verbal statements and actions like sarcasm and nasty comments about personal characteristics. In fact, if your partner is verbally aggressive, the likelihood of later physical violence is much increased. I believe that when verbal aggression is permitted to occur it is like a threshold has been crossed. Accepting some early forms of verbal abuse may communicate to your partner that this behavior is acceptable and opens the door to more of the same or worse as anger actions progress from the verbal to the physical.

It's time to take a close look at where you are on the slippery slope of anger and what you want to do about it. First take a look at the ladder depicted on the next page. Then review the list of risk factors for violence to see how many of these are present in your partner. When you add up all this information, you'll have a good idea of how urgent it is for you to take action right now. The rest of this chapter will then help you decide what actions to take, when, and how.

Realities of the Progression of Anger

- All of the behaviors on the ladder are poor ways of coping with and expressing anger. They are all inappropriate and likely to interfere with intimacy and effective communication.

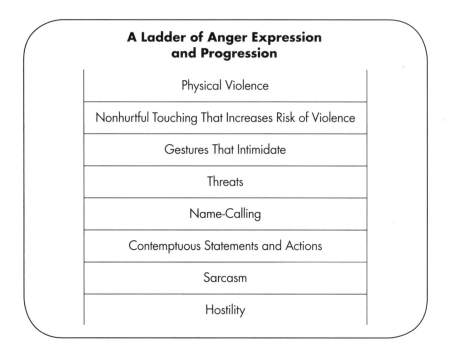

**A Ladder of Anger Expression
and Progression**

Physical Violence
Nonhurtful Touching That Increases Risk of Violence
Gestures That Intimidate
Threats
Name-Calling
Contemptuous Statements and Actions
Sarcasm
Hostility

- As anger expression becomes more aggressive, whether verbal or physical, the quality of your life will likely deteriorate.

- The more personally contemptuous of you your partner's anger expression becomes, the greater likelihood that your confidence, self-esteem, and general emotional health will be affected adversely.

- As your partner's anger actions escalate into the physical threats and actions described in this chapter, the risk of your being injured increases.

- Once any form of physical expression of anger is directed at you, including gestures without touching you (e.g., blocking your path, throwing things toward you), the likelihood of further physical abuse increases.

- If you are in any way touched in anger, the risk of being hurt increases dramatically and your safety is threatened.

Risk Factors for Violence

Much research has explored the personality, biological, and situational factors that increase the risk that a person will become violent. No *one* of these predicts violence, yet each has been associated with violence in the literature (Centers for Disease Control, 2008, Whitaker & Lutzker, 2009, O'Leary & Woodin, 2009). *Be aware that the most important risk factor by far is a history of past violence during the person's lifespan.* If your partner has never been violent to you or others, then the likelihood of future risk is reduced greatly.

How many of the following are present in your partner?

- *Past violence to partner or in intimate relationships*

  Risk increases if violence is:

  - More severe or causes injury
  - Frequent
  - Planned or deliberate
  - Occurring in other nonrelationship situations

- *Emotional or verbal abuse in current or past relationships*

- *Threats to harm self or others*

- *Victim of physical or emotional abuse in childhood*

- *Alcohol abuse or dependence; drug abuse*

- *Certain mental/emotional disorders (if untreated):*

  - Schizophrenia if accompanied by substance abuse
  - Paranoia/delusions that the person is being persecuted
  - Bipolar disorder

- *Severe personality disturbance or disorder that leads to instrumental expression of anger*

  - Psychopathy
  - Attachment-type personality disorders: borderline, narcissistic, histrionic, antisocial, or paranoid

- *High levels of poorly regulated anger or hostility*

- *Severe situational stress (e.g., job loss, financial stress)*

- *Attitudes supporting power and control or violence*

- *Presence of weapons*

Excuses, Excuses

Your partner might offer a variety of "reasons" for violent actions. Some may sound a bit legitimate, almost compelling. But don't be fooled: abuse by any description is inexcusable.

Have you heard any excuses that sound like these?

"If you had just listened to me and stopped talking, this [the abuse] wouldn't have happened."

"I didn't really mean to hit you; you just got in the way of my hand [fist, foot, flying object]. I was only trying to get your attention!"

"You must realize that this isn't me doing this—it's the incredible stress I've been under."

"If you could just leave before I get so mad, it would keep this from happening."

"I am so sorry. This is not me, and it won't happen ever again!"

"You do it too. What about the time you pushed me aside to get out of the house?"

Notice that each of these excuses puts the blame for the abusive actions on you or something else. It is *you* who caused it by being unreasonable or just not leaving soon enough, or it's "stress" and "not the real me" who is the culprit. These self-serving excuses are all aimed at trying to explain away an act that is intolerable under any circumstances other than for self-defense. Sadly, many partners try to believe these excuses and give their abusive partners chance after chance to reform.

WHAT TO DO WHEN ENOUGH IS ENOUGH

If you find yourself buying into your partner's excuses for violence, you may be reinforcing the very behavior that threatens your safety. The farther up the ladder you go, the more invasive the effects of inappropriate expressions of anger on you. And when it comes to verbal and physical aggression, perhaps it's easier said than done, but I believe you should tolerate NONE. PERIOD! Where are you on the ladder?

Start with Assessment (A)

Think about how you're reacting to your partner's behaviors that have put you somewhere on the ladder of escalating aggression. Review your RAP responses and Daily Log. How have you been responding to these behaviors up until now, and how has your approach seemed to impact your partner? Is aggression escalating?

Begin by identifying how you feel. Hunter had begun to feel increasingly anxious and worried that Charlotte's angry gestures would spin out of control. He also felt humiliated that she so often bullied him into conforming to what she wanted with her anger tactics. He told me he would often give in just to achieve peace. His actions other than placating her included editing what he said and did around her to avoid inciting an argument, particularly when she was "stressed out." Often he would redirect what he wanted to do or reschedule gatherings with friends and family if she gave him reason to believe she was not agreeable to the plans. While he said he wasn't afraid he'd be injured (she had never been physically violent to him or others), he did find himself doing everything he could think of to avoid the next escalation of anger. He was concerned about how out of control Charlotte might become and how he would cope without losing his own temper. Walking on eggshells was not working for him, and he felt he had tried "everything" to defuse her anger to no effect.

In contrast to Hunter, Lacey and Janice had in common a fear of their partners' explosive anger that had become physical in increasingly scary ways. Both reported that they had begun to dread any episode with their partners that led to conflict. Sam's acts of restraining her by holding her and blocking her movements led Lacey to feel more and more helpless, like a hostage to his rage. When he screamed in her face and "made" her listen to him, she felt like she was surrendering any sense of personal integrity and control of her life.

Janice had experienced threats and physically restrictive behaviors, as had Lacey, but lately Frank had begun to push her hard with his open hands and had hit her a few times while rationalizing it was not with his "closed fist." She was starting to worry about her safety; her husband might really hurt her. After all, he had already injured her back "by mistake," he said, when he pushed her and she fell backward across a table.

Frank also had significant risk factors: He had been violent in the past with others (he had once punched a neighbor whom he had accused of purposely making noise early in the morning and had a history of fights in high school and even in college). He had already been violent with Janice (despite his rationalizations that he had never "really" hit her with a closed fist). Frank also was a heavy "social" drinker who rarely got visibly intoxicated but was much more emotionally coiled and easily provoked when drinking. Many of his most frightening outbursts had occurred when he was drinking, even when he had had only two or three beers. He was likely to be clinically depressed, and his ability to manage his anger was poor, further increasing risk.

Where Are the Boundaries?

While both Lacey and Janice were frightened of their partners' anger and Janice now saw a significant risk of violence in Frank's past behavior, neither had yet set firm boundaries (B) for her partner. Both Lacey and Janice loved their partners and tended to mentally filter in the "good times" while ignoring episodes of aggression or rationalizing them away as "under too much stress" or "too much to drink." What to do? Both had been told to leave their partners by loved ones, but neither felt it was "bad enough" to separate and possibly rupture the relationship forever. Yet the status quo was unacceptable.

• **Unacceptable:** Each formulated a boundary that stated in no uncertain terms that NO threat of or act of unwanted physical touch or violence would be acceptable under any circumstances. There would be no exceptions to excuse their partners' mood, stresses, or anything else.

• **Acceptable:** Each made it clear that her partner was invited to express any ideas, suggestions, opinions, and all feelings, including anger and disappointment, in a calm and direct manner at a time that was mutually convenient. Janice and Lacey each modeled the "I" message format (Chapter 5) as they communicated and hoped their partners would copy it as an effective way to communicate with them.

What Beliefs Are Pulling the Strings?

For both Janice and Lacey the next step was to review their Daily Logs while keeping in mind what they now knew about their beliefs, or cognitions (C in our model; see Chapter 4). Each had her own unique thoughts about her partner's anger, but some version of the following—all common among those subjected to relationship aggression—was reported by one or both. These beliefs may block your efforts at asserting new boundaries. If you can identify with any of the ones shown in the table on the next page, write down the positive, fact-based counterbeliefs that come to mind or just start practicing affirming the "rational beliefs" in the right column.

Lacey wrote her new beliefs on a 3" × 5" card and placed it where she could see it everyday, which led her to read it and state one or more of the new beliefs several times a day. After a while the beliefs became her mantra, one or more restated in her mind whenever Sam even began to raise his voice. It empowered her to speak up early and stop his cascade into verbal and then physical aggression.

The Daily Logs of Janice, Hunter, and Lacey revealed that their self-talk was filled with cognitive distortions that reinforced their unhelpful beliefs and elicited overwhelming fear and hopelessness that made it impossible for them to think clearly. Here are some examples, with the cognitive distortions in **bold** type and the fact-based rebuttal below:

Lacey

- Situation: "Sam got so mad at me I couldn't believe it. He held me from leaving the living room until he had a chance to tell me how he felt. He held my arms and wouldn't let me go."

- Self-Talk (*Minimizing, Rationalizing*): "I hate it when he does that, but **he doesn't do this very often. He doesn't mean to hurt me**; he just gets so mad and wants me to stay and listen. I don't like it, but he loves me, and I guess **I have to understand he has a right to make me hear him out**."

- Rebuttal: "The fact is that any touch or restraint is abusive and I won't stand for it, no matter what he says."

Transforming Beliefs That Keep You from Asserting Your Boundaries

Unhelpful Beliefs	Rational Beliefs
"I'm powerless to change the situation I am in."	"I'm powerful and strong enough to stop any further violence."
"I can't handle my partner's anger."	"No matter what he/she does, I can handle it or find someone who can help me decide what to do."
"He/she is much stronger and will overwhelm me."	"I can and will stand up for myself and not tolerate anymore nasty comments or actions."
"Nothing seems to work to get him/her to change. It's hopeless."	"If I change my thinking, I know I can change things for me. I'm hopeful."
"My partner is abusive and may hurt me (or my children), so I better do what he/she wants."	"I am confident in myself and deserve to be treated with dignity, no matter what."
"I can't make it on my own, so I have to put up with it."	"I have coped with many challenges successfully, like when Dad died, and I will cope with this."
"Things will work out if I just give it enough time."	"Things will work out if I assert my boundaries and don't give in to my partner's threats."

Hunter

- Situation: "Charlotte got so angry she threatened to destroy our wedding picture, which I have always loved. I tried to calm her down."

- Self-Talk (*Rationalizing*): "**She can't help getting so angry after dealing with her clients all day. She brings in most of our income, and I have to realize that she deserves my understanding.**"

- Rebuttal: "The fact is that I deserve to be treated with dignity and not be abused no matter how much she earns or what stress she's under. I will let her know that her actions are over the top."

Janice

- Situation: "Frank threatened never to speak to my mother again if I didn't listen to his plea to go to his parents' house for Thanksgiving. When I disagreed, he put me down, calling me 'stupid' and 'bone-headed,' and later would not let me go to sleep until I agreed to do 'the right thing': give in to his 'totally reasonable' request. At one point he pulled the covers off the bed and started to pull me onto the floor to 'get me' to hear him."

- Self-Talk (*Tunnel Vision*): "I think this is wrong, but **he is usually such a good provider and good with the children.** I just cannot get him so furious that they will be frightened again. **I need to appreciate how good I have it: nice home, all the things I want, and happy kids. I can't complain, can I?**"

- Rebuttal: "He has no right to call me names or touch me in any way. I can have a truly good life only if I'm free from intimidation and abuse. I will not tolerate this."

Lacey

- Situation: "Sam got home from work and started yelling so loudly at the children that I was worried he would lose it and hit them."

- Self-Talk (*Self-Deprecating*): "Sam may lose it, **but who am I to complain too much? He married me knowing that I don't have a college degree like he does. He takes good care of me and doesn't seem to mind the weight I've gained. I really don't deserve to com-**

plain if he loses it sometimes. He doesn't really ever hit me, just threatens it when he's really mad."

• Rebuttal: "I choose to feel good about myself no matter what Sam thinks of me or my weight."

Each of these distortions fueled fear or in some way prevented them from asserting their perfect right to be free from any form of aggression or intimidation. As you look over your own Daily Log, what cognitive distortions can you identify that might be impeding your willingness to assert your new boundaries and stand up for what you believe with your partner? Remember, the sooner you can identify the roadblocks to asserting your rights as a partner and a person, the sooner your partner will have to confront your changes with a change of his or her own (or not, in which case you can decide to leave).

Denying Rewards and Expressing Expectations

If you're exposed to any form of physical aggression, you must now decide what you will do the next time this behavior occurs and stick to your course of action. Here are some rules of thumb suggested by multiple sources in the literature on violence between intimate partners:

1. *Any form of verbal aggression should not be tolerated.* Ever. Permitting your partner to treat you with contempt or name-calling greatly increases the risk that you will confront more serious abusive behavior in the future.

• *Options*: See Chapter 6.

2. *Even lesser forms of physical aggression, including threats, gestures that threaten without touch, any form of low-level physical gesture or touch that is unwanted, is totally unacceptable and an immutable part of your new boundary.*

• *Options*: Using an "I" message, take a firm stand that this behavior is intolerable and firmly ask your partner to stop immediately. Let your partner know in no uncertain terms that any future threat or touch, regardless of the reason for it, will not be tolerated, and you will immediately seek counseling and advice from experts and expect your partner to participate in the counseling. If this behavior recurs, let your partner know how you will handle it: separate from him or her for a period of time (e.g., 24 hours) or leave the house for a period of time. Again reit-

Researchers Arlene Weisz, Richard Tolman, and Daniel Saunders asked victims of violence how fearful they were of future aggression from their partners and found it was the best predictor of violence actually happening. If you're afraid of your partner (and only you can determine this), take your fear seriously and leave the situation. Get advice from a professional counselor about how to proceed.

erate that you expect your partner to seek counseling to address the underlying issues.

3. *Violent behavior that hurts or harms you is clearly unacceptable for any reason or under any circumstances, even if you are not seriously injured.* Permitting acts of physical violence to occur without serious consequences greatly increases the likelihood that you will be injured in the future. Almost all professional advice you would receive from clinicians and researchers would tell you to call 911 to get help immediately to ensure your safety or **leave the situation immediately or as soon as it is safe to do** (with any children) for your safety and protection. The Suggested Resources section at the back of the book lists numerous websites and telephone numbers of agencies and organizations that provide direct services to you, like access to women's shelters and hotlines for immediate help, as well as many books and materials to be found online to educate yourself on your options. In all cases I recommend that you seek counseling and discuss with your counselor if and when to bring your partner into the therapy.

Hunter and Charlotte

Hunter decided to use strong "I" messages to tell Charlotte that threatening him, throwing objects, destroying things, and using any other intimidating (if noncontact) gestures would no longer be allowed.

> CHARLOTTE: (*In a fit of anger, throws a glass in Hunter's direction and threatens to smash more.*) I hate you! You never make me feel loved. All you do is work, and you're obsessed with your job. Why don't you just live at the office?! I would never miss you—that's for sure!
>
> HUNTER: You just threw a glass at me. I am totally confused and

frustrated that you can't seem to talk about your feelings without resorting to threatening me in some way. I want to listen but can't get beyond the violence. Could we talk in a calm voice and give each other a chance to express what we feel without interrupting or getting physical? I would really appreciate that. You should know that I will immediately stop the conversation and leave the room or the house anytime you become physical by throwing or smashing or if you call me names. Once things calm down, I am always willing to talk in a calm voice about what you and I need from each other. What do you think?

Notice that Hunter talks only about how *he* feels and what *he* thinks and needs, without showing any contempt for or criticism of Charlotte. He makes clear where his boundaries are and yet expresses a willingness to talk, provided talk is calm and without interruptions. Hunter soon realizes that he does indeed have the power to decide what he is willing to participate in and what he is not willing to do. It feels good. Soon Charlotte begins to avoid raising her voice and threatening Hunter with throwing things because it gets her no acknowledgment of her needs. When she begins to raise her voice or threaten Hunter in any way, he immediately tells her that he is about to stop the discussion and leave the situation until she can communicate in a calm way. When her old behaviors of threatening him no longer work in any way, she abandons them and tries to sit down and talk in a calm way to get Hunter's attention. What works is what she ends up doing, which is true of most of us. Hunter also suggested couple counseling for the two and makes it clear that he will attend by himself if necessary if the two cannot begin to talk things out without aggression.

In contrast, Lacey and Janice had been touched in anger by their partners, which greatly increases the risk of further violence. Both felt intimidated when their partners acted out their anger with holding, blocking, slapping, or shoving. Both had decided that such behaviors were unacceptable and would not be tolerated in the future. The issue was how to communicate this and how their partners would react if they took a stand. Would they be hurt in some way, and what if their partners decided to leave them? All of these fears had paralyzed them up until now.

Both Lacey and Janice decided that *no touch of any kind* would be tolerated in the future. Both decided to work out a plan to separate from their partners if any further incident of aggression occurred. The Suggested Resources at the end of this book offer support and specific strategies for developing a "Safety Planning List" of specific items you should set aside or address so you are ready to leave the situation immediately if physical violence occurs again or for any reason you fear for your safety.

Lacey and Janice, like Hunter, used the "I" message approach to make it clear that any further touching in anger, for any reason, was unacceptable and would be met with separation: either their partners would be asked to leave or they would leave. Both agreed that if they were injured or felt their partners wouldn't let them leave the home they would call 911 and report the situation. Neither wanted to call the police, but both soon realized that their safety and that of their children was the top priority. The literature on coping with physical abuse suggests that you must take a bold step to clearly communicate that abusive actions will no longer be tolerated in the future, before the next situation arises, as well as immediately should it happen.

Lacey and Sam

LACEY: (*In response to Sam refusing to let her leave the bedroom by blocking and holding her until he had his "say."*) I will not tolerate your holding or touching me in any way to keep me a captive so you can talk. Let go or I will pack up and leave as soon as I get out of here. I will no longer be your hostage.

SAM: (*Lets go and permits Lacey to leave the room.*) Come on. This isn't a big deal. I didn't really hurt you, did I? Get a life!

LACEY: It's a big deal to me. We may be arguing, and I wish we wouldn't. But there is no reason to call me names and touch me like you do sometimes. I have a right to ask you to stop and to leave. If this behavior occurs again, I am leaving and will only return when I feel safe. Also, I will call a counselor to learn how to better deal with your anger and our issues. I would hope you would go also.

About a week after Lacey set her boundary with Sam, he began putting down her intelligence and calling her "stupid" and "foolish" when she disagreed with his intention to buy a new car. As was often the case, the discussion began peacefully and escalated when the two disagreed about what they could afford. Both began to raise their voices, and Lacey decided things were getting too intense and told Sam she was going to call a "STOP" (recall the defusing strategies from Chapter 5) to end the conversation and leave until she calmed down; she invited him to do the same. He refused to stop talking and followed her when she retreated to their bedroom. When she again asked him to stop, he told her she was being unfair and refused to leave. When Lacey started to leave the room, he blocked her passage and held on to her arms to restrain her from leaving.

> SAM: (*Yelling at Lacey.*) Just wait a minute. Let me speak! There's no way you're leaving until you listen to me. I have a right to be heard! (*Blocks Lacey from going to the bedroom door, then holds on to her arm.*)
>
> LACEY: Let go immediately. This is abusive, and I won't stand for it. (*Using the "broken record" defusing strategy, keeps calmly and firmly repeating "Please let go" and refuses to talk with Sam about the issue until he finally releases her and she leaves the room.*)

Lacey immediately got the bag she had already packed and left the house to go to a friend's home. She called Sam to let him know she was all right and would be home when she felt ready. She also contacted me and set up an appointment to discuss what had happened and her options. When Lacey returned home two days later, she made it clear that the next time any touch occurred she would be gone until she had clear evidence he had begun counseling and was sincerely working on his anger. Once they were together again, Sam decided to come into counseling and began to address his anger issues along the lines outlined in my book *Taking Charge of Anger*. Both decided to enter couple counseling with the goal of staying together.

Now that Lacey had stood up for her boundaries, Sam began to correct himself when he started down the road of verbal aggression or any touching of her in anger. For example, he would start to hold on to her and then let go, saying "I'm sorry, but when you're ready, can we talk?" He soon learned that Lacey must agree to talk and that he could not "make" her talk with him. Because he loved her and wanted the relationship to work, he was motivated to make changes. Unfortunately, this will not always be the case. Setting your boundaries is still critical, though. Your boundaries set the stage for your partner to make changes or not, as he or she so desires. But they preserve your own safety and security.

Janice and Frank

Janice decided that Frank's hitting and shoving was already excessive and resolved that she would call the police if he ever hit her again, no matter what the consequences for Frank. Frank often insisted that his anger was beyond his control and that if she notified anyone his reputation would be destroyed or he might be fired. Janice had so far avoided talking about her plight with anyone for fear that Frank would be hurt by the revelation. After talking with me and reading some of the resources I suggested, she decided to attend a group for battered women offered by the local YWCA and to continue working on improving her self-esteem and ability to assert her boundaries with her husband. She had encouraged Frank to find his own therapist to address his rage and violence, but he refused, telling her that he knew he had a problem but had to learn to cope with it "on my own. I don't believe in therapists!"

> JANICE: (*Finds a time when she has Frank's full attention. Calmly approaches him.*) Frank, last night you again pushed me onto the bed. You already injured my back a few weeks ago when you pushed me, even though I know you didn't want me to fall on that table. This makes me feel very hurt, sad, and very angry at you and myself that I have put up with this as long as I have. That's over! I am letting you know that the next time you touch me in any way when angry, no matter what your excuse, I am calling the police to report it and I am leaving. I won't return until you are in counseling and have made enough progress that I can feel safe. If not, I won't return at all.

> FRANK: (*obviously stunned and surprised*) What do you mean you're calling the police? My job is at stake here! You wouldn't embarrass me like that, would you? I have never really tried to hurt you; you know that.

> JANICE: It doesn't matter what you haven't 'tried' to do; you have physically abused me and hurt me in many ways, and I will never tolerate it again. If you don't want to be embarrassed, don't touch me. It's that simple. I am not kidding and will do what I say.

> FRANK: Couldn't you be more reasonable? What if I lose my job? I love you and don't want to lose you! Don't do this.

JANICE: That's exactly how I feel: I love you too, Frank, and I wish you wouldn't do this to me. If you touch me again, I will follow through!

To her credit, Janice followed through when Frank got furious a few weeks later and grabbed her shoulders, shaking her to "get her to come to her senses." He was again shocked and dismayed when Janice got on the phone and called the police, who came to the house and interviewed both of them. While they didn't arrest Frank, they made a report and let him know that the next time they would arrest him since Janice feared for her safety. They did recommend that he leave the house, which he did, and Janice told him he could not return (he stayed with a brother) until he got into counseling for his anger and she and the therapist felt things were safe. In addition to his counseling, Janice agreed to enter couple therapy to work with him on improving their communication and how they discussed differences. Janice felt very empowered by taking a stand with Frank and felt confident she would now do whatever it took to ensure she would never again be physically abused. For his part Frank seemed to be happy that things had changed when I met with the two of them a few months later. He reported that meeting with his therapist had been helpful not only in resolving his anger but in communicating with his peers at work and with his adult children.

WHEN TO SEEK PROFESSIONAL HELP?

The stories of Charlotte and Hunter, Lacey and Sam, and Janice and Frank may make it seem pretty simple to intervene when physical aggression rears its head in your relationship. I'm sure you already know it's not that easy. These couples experienced lots of ups and downs on their way to making their relationships work better for all concerned, and all of them took advantage of some type of professional advice or counseling, either individually or as a couple. Chapter 6 discusses medical and psychological problems your partner may be experiencing that contribute to unhelpful anger expression and that make a referral for evaluation and/ or treatment advisable. In addition to individual treatment for your partner, couple counseling is often beneficial. (See the Suggested Resources at the end of the book for more information.)

You're probably wondering yourself when counseling is wise. Ask yourself these questions:

1. Are you finding success in understanding and implementing the ideas in this book on your own? If so, carry on. You probably have a lot of emotional and psychological awareness to begin with and may do very well by applying what you have learned here and from the other readings.

2. Do you feel overwhelmed with your partner's anger and find these ideas overwhelming also? Or perhaps you are not having success applying new boundaries and seem to run into serious roadblocks (see Chapter 10) with your partner. If it seems difficult to surmount problems in communicating or resolving relationship issues, couple counseling may provide you with the guidance to break out of old patterns into the kind of relationship you've always desired. Select someone who is an appropriately licensed mental health counselor and who has experience in working with conflict, anger, and abuse in relationships.

3. If you have identified with this chapter and find yourself with a partner who is physically violent, you are frightened for your safety, or your relationship seems way too intense or scary lately, seek professional counseling for yourself immediately. You may decide or your counselor may suggest that you separate from your partner right away given the current situation. Also, counseling groups offered by local agencies can be of great comfort and help.

WHEN ANGER IS AGGRESSIVE YET PASSIVE

So far we have been describing anger that is overt and expressed in ways that are hard to misinterpret. It's clear that when your partner is yelling at you, making a sarcastic remark, or using some form of verbal aggression he or she is in fact angry. The emotion is unmistakable and leads directly to questions about why this is happening and what you can do to make it stop. But sometimes you may find yourself wondering what your partner *is* feeling. Is it anger or something else? When anger is indirect or passive, you can end up feeling offended, hurt, or assaulted, but still wondering if your reaction is appropriate to the situation. Your partner may withhold something you would like or have asked for. Or perhaps she or he stops talking and avoids any discussion, spending time alone or lost in thought. You try to discuss what is obviously wrong and get a reply like "Why, nothing. I'm fine." Yet you know things are not right and you hope that eventually he or she will reveal what is wrong.

Remember John and Nancy from Chapter 1? Nancy would often meet John with an "icy" greeting when he arrived home late from being out with his friends. If she was angry, she might spend the rest of the evening in their bedroom, ignoring him and then not talking for days at a time. This cold anger was very provocative to John and just as upsetting to him as some of the more intense faces of anger were to others you've read about.

The next chapter describes these indirect expressions of "passive" anger and offers ways of using the A–E model to set a different kind of boundary for behavior that sometimes is not clearly angry but is always confusing and challenging.

9

PASSIVE ANGER

What to Do When It *Seems* Harmless but *Feels* Harmful

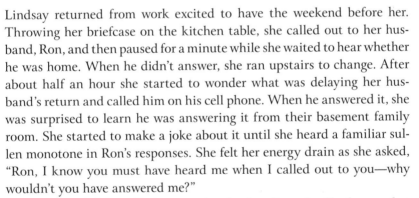

Lindsay returned from work excited to have the weekend before her. Throwing her briefcase on the kitchen table, she called out to her husband, Ron, and then paused for a minute while she waited to hear whether he was home. When he didn't answer, she ran upstairs to change. After about half an hour she started to wonder what was delaying her husband's return and called him on his cell phone. When he answered it, she was surprised to learn he was answering it from their basement family room. She started to make a joke about it until she heard a familiar sullen monotone in Ron's responses. She felt her energy drain as she asked, "Ron, I know you must have heard me when I called out to you—why wouldn't you have answered me?"

Lindsay didn't really listen to her husband's reply. She knew what he'd say: "I *didn't* hear you—I was watching the game. Why do you make such a big deal out of everything?" or "I *would* have answered if I'd actually heard you. Why would you accuse me of purposely ignoring you?" or "I'm just watching the game. If you wanted to see me, why didn't you come down here?"

Why would Ron withdraw to the basement or refuse to acknowledge his wife's arrival home? Why is Lindsay almost expecting that Ron won't reply honestly about his feelings? The fact is that Ron is still angry

183

at Lindsay for being too tired to respond to his sexual advances the night before. When Ron is angry, he typically does not come right out and discuss his feelings or their origin. He grew up in a family where no one ever revealed their true feelings but would suffer in silence, refusing to talk for days at a time to get their point across or to make the object of their anger suffer. Lindsay has become used to this and has almost given up trying to get Ron to talk about his emotions. She was never sure what she could have done to make him angry. All she knew was that he treated her as if she was responsible for whatever was bugging him but wouldn't tell her what that was or how she could make it better. She'd end up either sitting in silence with him or retreating to another room feeling terribly lonely, frustrated that her husband had turned the "problem" on her.

Typically Lindsay would start out asking Ron directly if something was wrong. He'd invariably say something to this effect: "No. Why do you always think the worst? I'm fine. I just need my space." If she questioned him again, he'd accuse her of nagging him or of being insecure—suggesting that she was the one with the problem.

The outward, more direct, intense forms of anger discussed in previous chapters can throw you off balance by leaving you feeling blamed for your partner's displeasure or frustration. But the passive type of anger that Lindsay's husband typically expressed can leave the recipient even more confused. Like Lindsay, you may question not just why your partner is so angry but even *whether* your partner is angry. Is your reading of the behavior accurate? Your reaction to your partner's behavior may leave little doubt that he or she is angry at you—or at someone or something else and is taking it out on you. But when your partner completely denies being angry and is not behaving in an outwardly aggressive way, you can feel as if you're being "gaslighted"—tricked into self-doubt to the point where you start questioning your perceptions.

At the very least, passive–aggressive faces of anger can make you feel dejected and helpless. You're being treated as if you're an offender, the perpetrator of some transgression, but also cut off from communication and denied any opportunity to make up for or correct whatever you must have done. Little else can make you feel so helpless.

PASSIVE ANGER HAS TWO FACES

Lindsay's husband, Ron, withheld what she wanted by "forgetting" to fulfill her requests, talking to her as little as possible, not being affectionate, and sometimes ignoring her for periods of time as a way of expressing his anger. This is one of two faces of passive anger—what you have often heard called **passive–aggression**.The other involves just turning off and withdrawing from you, which I call **cold anger**.

Harry would pout but deny he was upset or angry. His passive anger was often fueled when Grace would criticize him for something or offer a suggestion about how he could do it "better." For example, Harry installed a shelf in the pantry at Grace's request to provide more storage for their food items. He felt good about what he had done, but when Grace got home from work she immediately went to the pantry and commented that the shelf was too small and not centered properly on the wall. Harry's self-talk was immediately filled with inner comments like "No matter what I do, she finds fault with it," and "I can't take any more put-downs when I'm doing the best I can for her and our family." These negative thoughts remained in his head as he never discussed his feelings of hurt and resentment with Grace so they could be resolved ("What's the use? She won't listen anyway!"). Instead, he would pout and fume to himself, then act out his anger in one of the passive ways just discussed. That had been his style when angry since he was a child in a home where he was never permitted to express his emotions. Because these resentments were not resolved, he carried them around with him and became all the more sensitive to any critical remarks. Thus it seemed he was unapproachable and distant much of the time.

> **Passive anger** includes a host of behaviors that **withhold, withdraw,** or in some indirect way create discomfort for the other person, **without actively identifying or expressing the underlying anger.**

When Grace reached out to hug him, he would often stiffen or pull away. When she did something special for him, he would barely comment on it or would pick on some minor flaw: "This pie crust is kind of tough"; "But when you called the airline for me, did you ask about upgrades?" He would thus "pay her back" through an ineffective way of acting out his resentment. Grace felt punished by these passive actions, but Harry would never admit he was angry, purposely withholding from her. Grace felt she had to become a mind reader to try to figure out what Harry was feeling and wanting from her or the relationship. Given that she couldn't find a course to take called "Mind Reading 101," she was stuck with ambiguity and limited information to decide how to react to her husband. Harry maintained that he had "no problems"—the only problem for him was Grace's "nagging."

Grace knew their relationship was suffering because of whatever Harry was so unhappy about. She was frustrated and unhappy because almost none of her needs were being met while Harry spent so much time withdrawing from her. She just couldn't have a personal conversation with her husband, yet they remained in a kind of "Holy Deadlock." Grace was ready to leave, but held on to the dream that Harry would change. "Some relationship with him is better than no relationship, I guess," was Grace's half-hearted rationale for staying with him.

- *Passive anger is a vicious circle.* One of the most destructive aspects of passive anger is that it creates a vicious circle that can feel almost impossible to break out of. Ron meant more to Lindsay than anyone else in her life, and yet she couldn't get him to tell her what was wrong. So she persisted in trying to find out. When she repeatedly asked him, she was labeled as the "problem" ("Why are you nagging me? *Nothing is wrong!* Why can't you just leave well enough alone and stop complaining all the time?"). Being characterized unfairly in this way naturally made her feel hurt and angry herself. The frustration and aggravation she felt has a way of driving people to find the answer they need, and so Lindsay kept trying to get Ron to talk—which led him to withdraw more and accuse her more and more of nagging.

- *Being passive and aggressive is a contradiction.* Without words it communicates "I am angry with you, but I won't act angry, nor will I admit to my true feelings and thoughts. Instead, I will do something you don't want or not do something you want me to do to punish you, but deny that's what I'm doing."

- *Your partner's passive anger may be even harder for you to cope with than outward anger, even of the inappropriate kind.* When your partner is intensely angry, visibly and audibly, at least you know what's going on and can set your boundaries accordingly. Passive anger, on the other hand, is often difficult to identify. You might feel instinctually very certain that your partner is angry without having any evidence to support your claim. And, unfortunately, most people who resort to passive–aggression will go to great lengths to refute any proof you try to present. If you can't put your finger on what your partner is doing that you object to, and/or your partner simply denies doing it, how can you define and enforce a specific boundary?

All of this can leave you feeling at sea, completely unsure of your ability to judge your partner's behavior—or your reaction to it. The following indications may help give you an anchor from which to regain your self-confidence:

A LITMUS TEST FOR PASSIVE ANGER

If your partner engages in the following types of behavior, you're probably on the receiving end of passive anger:

• *Withholding praise, attention, or positive feedback from you when you deserve or ask for it.* For example, Harry rarely praised Grace, even when she went out of her way to please him. Grace felt Harry seemed to enjoy her struggles to earn his kind words.

• *"Forgetting" or failing to follow through when a request is made* ("Please pick up the dry cleaning"; "Would you straighten up the living room, please?"), so that you end up feeling frustrated, confused, or annoyed. In *Living with the Passive–Aggressive Man*, Scott Wetzler called this tendency "fostering chaos," which means your partner "prefers to leave the puzzle incomplete, the job undone," negatively impacting your options and choices. Sometimes Ron would "forget" to give Lindsay an important telephone message that would then rob her of the opportunity to get together with her close friends.

• *"Stalling" when you want to discuss an issue you've identified, thus blocking resolution of the issue.*

• *Responding to your needs for affection by withholding intimacy.* Harry, for example, would often go to bed early when upset with Grace, thus avoiding any closeness.

• *Engaging in behavior that is known to upset you and then denying any negative motives.* Examples might include preparing a disliked meal, painting the wrong shutters, leaving newspapers all over the living room, "forgetting" to give you the car keys, smoking a cigarette around you when your partner knows you have allergies and you have asked him or her not to.

• *Being chronically late to activities when clearly aware this upsets you.* As your partner dawdles and procrastinates far beyond almost anyone else's limit of patience, opportunities are lost and time is squandered. But even more fundamentally important to the passive–aggressive partner, apparently, is that lateness says this relationship will be run on his or her schedule, by his or her rules and standards, not yours.

• *Responding to your questions about his or her significant thoughts, feelings, and needs with a minimal response* (e.g., "Whatever!"; "I don't know"; "Fine!"; "Forget about it") when it is clear from your partner's actions that something is wrong.

Tell yourself that if you've seen this behavior in your partner, you're not imagining it. Remember that your passively angry partner will likely deny anger and give a perfectly reasonable explanation for actions that frustrate and confuse you. But it can be maddening even when you confirm that you're seeing what you think you're seeing, because you still don't understand why it's happening. Is your partner angry and getting even? Is this a way to communicate a message that you just have to interpret correctly to understand? Can you really be sure your partner isn't honestly expressing a preference or isn't really surprised at your reaction? You're bound to question yourself; after all, this is the person you've come to trust as much as we usually trust anyone in our lives. Why would he or she act this way and then deny it? Let's take a look at that question:

Why Does Your Partner Act This Way?

While it's beyond the scope of this book to review all the speculations and theories about why some of us adopt a passive way of expressing anger, having an overview of the kinds of childhood experiences that seem most likely to contribute to the passive anger of the adult can help dispel some of your confusion about your partner's aggravating behavior. In *Overcoming Passive–Aggression*, Tim Murphy and Loriann Oberlin reviewed six possible explanations for what they call "hidden anger." No one factor is likely to explain why your partner is passively angry, but one or more of these may likely contribute to this frustrating pattern. The sidebar on the next page describes each of these factors. From your knowledge of your partner's childhood, which of these seems to make sense?

Clearly, passive anger may have its roots in a life script learned in the distant past, a script that now directs how the person thinks, feels, and acts when confronted by conflict. If you're aware of your partner's having been affected by any of the factors in the sidebar, you have further evidence that what you're witnessing is in fact passive anger. But if you still have any doubts, you can use the following questions as a guide.

Childhood Experiences May Contribute to Hidden Anger

Hidden Anger That Protects: Your partner may have learned and still uses "defense mechanisms" like these that protected him/her from punishment, parental anger, or pain.

- **Blaming** ("It wasn't me. It's your fault!")

- **Denial** ("Not true. I didn't do it.")

- **Repression** ("I just don't want to discuss it.")

- **Covering up important feelings** (It's okay. I don't mind.")

Hidden Anger as a Reaction: Your partner was exposed to physical, emotional, or sexual abuse and learned to hold his or her feelings inside out of fear of more abuse if he or she revealed what was going on. Also, hidden anger may be the result of sudden change (such as a new sister, a move) that impacted your partner and that your partner did not risk expressing.

Hidden Anger Searching for a Close Personal Bond: If your partner failed to develop a close attachment to parents or other childhood caregivers, he or she may not have learned how to form close relationships or trust enough to express inner feelings and so now has problems with expressing emotions and being intimate.

Hidden Anger as a Learned Behavior: Your partner learned from the actions of parents who never openly discussed emotions, dismissed "feelings," or failed to work out differences in front of the children. This learning could leave your partner unwilling and/or unable to open up.

Based on T. Murphy and L. H. Oberlin (2005). *Overcoming passive–aggression: How to stop hidden anger from spoiling your relationships, career and happiness.* New York: Wiley.

When, Where, and How Often Does Passive Anger Occur?

1. *How often does your partner withdraw or withhold?* Occasionally disagreeing with you or forgetting to pick up something from the store once in a blue moon should hardly get your attention. This seems perfectly normal. But when you notice that you are frequently met with a "No, I'm fine!" when it seems clear your partner isn't fine, or you have to put

up with lateness so often your complaints are beginning to sound like a broken record, you should be prepared to confront this misbegotten expression of anger.

2. *What is the context and history of your partner's passive actions?* Does this behavior occur in a particular kind of situation (such as soon after you've said or done something your partner doesn't like or after your partner's facial expression or tone of voice clearly indicates upset)? Of course, you have to be careful you are not merely "mind-reading" a feeling that is not present, but over time these patterns are likely to become clear. For example, Ron would often withdraw from Lindsay's efforts at talking and sometimes retreat to the bedroom to be alone ("cold anger") whenever she confronted him about his not trying to help around the house. He was angry because he felt he already did enough by going to a job every day and resented her "demands" he help out, but he would not state this clearly. They both worked full-time jobs and were forced to do most housework on the weekends. Ron would often "forget" to do an assigned task or do the job so poorly Lindsey had to redo it. Lindsay realized he was being manipulative with his passive anger, and she often fell for it. Her own resentment at his lack of participation and withdrawal from her and his unwillingness to go to counseling to improve himself and the relationship left her frustrated and in a kind of limbo.

3. *Do you increasingly find the quality of your life deteriorating as you confront your partner's passive tactics?* Are you often resentful or frustrated, or do you just feel resigned to putting up with a relationship that is not as fulfilling as it once was? These recurring feelings should not be discounted in your quest to try to make things better.

FROM PASSIVE TO ACTIVE: PULLING THE FOUNDATION OUT FROM UNDER PASSIVE–AGGRESSIVE TACTICS

A person who expresses anger passively will not change until he or she can admit it's a problem and learn to communicate feelings clearly and directly. This may very well require the help of a counselor. Meanwhile, though, you may reach the point where you must change to make things change for you. Living with a passively angry partner creates significant stress, fueled by a lack of control over your destiny. You are uncertain what the problem is in the most important relationship of your life. You can't make things better because you're not really sure what needs to change. Sometimes this lack of predictability and low sense of control creates anxiety that can impact your energy level, efficiency in getting things done, and self-confidence. Even your health can suffer, as pointed out in Chapter 2.

Grace began to feel it was hopeless to get Harry to open up and clearly express his feelings when he was upset with her. She had tried pleading with him, berating his passiveness, shaming him (e.g., "You can't even step up like a man and say what you want. You are a poor excuse for a husband!"), and placating him ("Okay, Harry. You win—what do you want?"). In response he would stay withdrawn until *he* decided to be responsive again. Sometimes his passive anger would last for days at a time. Grace finally decided to reconsider her relationship with Harry after she spent a weekend feeling alone while sitting right next to him. She was aware that he was angry with her but not sure why. He avoided conversation, wouldn't open up about his feelings, and passively gave in to whatever she requested while showing no interest in any of it.

GRACE: Harry, let's get out of here. Want to go to a movie?

HARRY: That's Okay. Whatever ... okay, if you want to.

GRACE: Harry, no, it's not going to be fun if you're not really into it.

HARRY: No, I'll go (*sighing and turning away*). Just let me finish this chapter (*reading and occasionally glancing at Grace*).

GRACE: So, Harry, are you upset about something? Why are you so unenthusiastic about anything I suggest?

HARRY: What do you mean? I'm not upset. Why do you have to always make such a big deal about everything? I'm fine. You're the one who obviously has a problem.

GRACE: (*sighing loudly*) I give up, Harry. Fine! Just read your book and stay as cold and distant as you want.

HARRY: Get a grip. You've started another argument again. You can never be happy. (*Looks at his book and continues reading.*)

GRACE: (*Walks away.*)

Like Harry, Ron often hid his underlying feelings or opinions, but unlike Harry, Ron would either postpone or abandon tasks he'd agreed to do until Lindsay lost all patience. "Ron, why are you doing this to me?" Lindsay asked him over and over. "I count on you, and you don't follow through. Why can't you just do one thing thoroughly? All I ask is that you finish what you start."

Rules of Thumb for Changing *Your* Script in the Face of Passive Anger

If you, like Lindsay and Grace, have decided that your partner is indeed engaging in passive anger and you are frustrated and confused by these indirect behaviors, what can you do to take charge of your own responses and thus improve your life in the relationship? Here are some guidelines:

• **Stop demanding that your partner admit to being angry and demand change in specific objectionable behaviors instead.** You're not a mind reader, and even if your interpretation of what lies beneath your partner's behavior is accurate, demanding an admission only rewards withholding/withdrawing behaviors by giving in to what your partner may want. Perhaps your partner wants to punish you, confuse you (e.g., don't take me for granted), or express dissatisfaction/anger at your behavior or his or her own dependency/inadequacy. For example, Grace would often plead with Harry to talk to her, usually to no avail:

GRACE: Why won't you just tell me how you feel and what you want from me? If you would please open up, I think we could be happier.

HARRY: (*looking away*) I don't know what you're talking about. I talk with you all the time. Stop blaming me for everything!

GRACE: Harry, please be honest with me.

HARRY: Don't you ever stop? (*Walks into the next room, sits down, and begins reading the newspaper.*)

When Lindsay asked Ron what he wanted to do over the coming weekend, she got no further than Grace:

RON: (*Sighs.*) *You* decide, as usual. I really don't care. Just let me know what we're doing.

LINDSAY: What's the matter? You seem upset with me. Have I made you mad somehow?

RON: I'm fine. I'm not angry. I just don't really care where we go.

LINDSAY: I know you're angry and you won't admit it.

Here's what Lindsay could have said instead, using an "I" message:

LINDSAY: I feel very frustrated right now because you won't tell me how you would like to spend this weekend. I would appreciate your telling me exactly what you would like to do so I can consider it and we can craft a plan. I will listen and do my best to accommodate you. Just tell me what you think so I can consider it.

RON: (*not giving up his withholding easily*) I'm fine. I really am okay with you deciding.

LINDSAY: Well, I can't force you to open up with me, but I want to hear your ideas and needs when you're ready. Until then, I'll make a plan and you can come or not.

• **In no way discourage your partner from expressing his or her feelings directly.** Do you ever say "I don't want to hear it" or "Why are you so upset? Get over it" when your partner *does* express anger or criticism directly? If so, you may be forcing him or her to go underground into passive faces of anger. Just insist that this expression be direct or you will not attend to it.

• **Avoid retaliation in any form.** While it's understandable to feel resentment and to want to retaliate, doing so just gives your partner a justification to continue passive anger. When Lindsay tried to have a direct discussion with Ron about helping out with the children, he refused to give his full attention to her ideas. She reached a boiling point of frustration and unloaded her anger on him, which is clearly not helpful.

RON: You decide. I'm trying to read my magazine. Can't you see that?

LINDSAY: I have been trying to discuss the kids with you all day, and you keep putting me off. When will you talk?

RON: What's the point? You'll just do what you do anyway. You don't really care about my opinions. I'm just the meal ticket here, not the father.

LINDSAY: That's ridiculous! I'm trying to get your ideas, and you won't even talk with me.

RON: Do we have to do this now? You always pick a time when I'm already doing something. You're so selfish.

LINDSAY: (*raising her voice*) You are a disgrace as a father and as a husband. I can't count on you to do anything. If you just avoid me, I'll end up doing it all, right? You make me sick! (*Stomps off and slams the bedroom door.*)

RON: (*Smiles and shakes his head, yells after her.*) I knew you would end up yelling again and putting me down. I just can't talk to you.

• **Identify your feelings and what you would appreciate in the future.** Again, use "I" messages, such as "I feel very dismissed and sad when you won't tell me how you're feeling. I'd really appreciate it if you would just tell me how you feel." Be clear and descriptive and avoid pejorative labels, like calling your partner cold, dismissive, manipulative, or passive–aggressive.

• **Be clear about what you expect from now on and also what you will no longer do.** Make clear that you will be happy to listen to any direct statements your partner makes about his or her thoughts, feelings, or needs. You expect your partner to be direct and complete in telling you what he or she is willing to do or not do and to communicate angry feelings immediately in a respectful manner, such as by using "I" messages.

You will also no longer make heroic efforts to figure out what your partner "really" means. Instead, you will take what he or she says—"I really don't want to talk," "I am not hungry"—at face value and not try to become a mind reader, asking questions like "Are you mad at me?" and "Do you resent something?" and "Are you afraid of what I will do?"

You will not become a kind of therapist trying to "psychologize" about your partner's unmet and unexpressed needs, speculating in this way: "I guess you won't talk with me because deep down you are unhappy and scared. This is probably because your mom is so critical. Does that make sense?"

You will no longer make excuses—"I guess she's just too overwhelmed to remember to pick up the dry cleaning for me"; "His job is really stressful, and I can't expect him to pitch in around here"—when your partner fails to do a fair share of the emotional or physical work of the relationship. Instead, if your partner "forgets" to do something agreed on, you'll clearly convey that this is unacceptable.

• **Let your partner experience the logical and natural consequences of his or her passive tactics.** Here are some examples to illustrate the concept. The real-world outcomes are in *italics*:

He failed to pick up his dry cleaning, so *let him be without a clean shirt*.

She won't tell you where she wants to go that evening, so *you decide where to go and invite a close friend to go with you*.

He won't tell you how he feels, so *you ignore any further discussion or antics until he is willing to speak up and tell you his inner feelings* (e.g., "Okay, I'll have to assume you'll let me know when you're ready to talk. I won't ask you again"). *You make your decisions without regard to how he might feel if he won't be forthcoming.* For example, Grace might say: "Harry, I've asked you for your opinion or feelings. Since you won't open up, I'll make the decision that suits me."

She won't speak to you and retreats to another part of the house. You let her know you wish she would be with you but that it's her choice. *You will go on with your day or evening, doing what pleases you without regard to her until she is willing to approach you directly.* For example, Grace learned to meet Harry's cold anger by saying something like "If you don't wish to be with me, Harry, I will go on with my own plans. I've decided to go to dinner with my sister. Have a nice evening."

USING THE A–E MODEL WITH PASSIVE ANGER

Keen Awareness That Leads to New Boundaries (A and B)

When Lindsay reviewed her RAP and Daily Log, she quickly realized how incredibly angry and hopeless she felt. She recognized that she often edited her thoughts and actions when around Ron—trying to "reduce his stress" so he wouldn't withdraw from conversation. Whenever she wanted to ask Ron to pitch in around the house or do her a small favor, she found herself thinking "How do I say this to him so he won't get mad?" or "What can I do to make things calmer for him?" Sometimes she found herself redirecting conversation and activities away from anything that might set off his irritation and then withdrawal. The more he withdrew from her, the more anxious she became, until she couldn't stand it and found herself refusing to answer his questions. Upon reflection Lindsay decided that meeting Ron's withdrawal from her with a kind of counterwithdrawal was not an effective solution: it didn't cause Ron to change and only made her feel less in control of herself.

As her recognition of the current situation grew, she became aware of the imbalance in their relationship. Ron managed to elicit intense feelings in his wife by doing very little—a hallmark of passive anger. His words were minimal, his actions were defined more by what he didn't do than by what he did do, and his response was basically "I'm fine—you're the one with the problem." With little effort Ron was evoking intense emotions and actions within Lindsay and then turning them against her: "Why are you so upset? You really are too sensitive and emotional."

> Passive anger creates a serious imbalance in a relationship: your partner uses minimal words and actions to evoke intense emotions in you—and then holds them against you.

Grace also reported feeling that she did all the heavy emotional "lifting" in the relationship and that Harry's minimal commitment to communication left her feeling hurt and resentful—but to no avail. It seemed that Harry wasn't about to change. In fact Harry's passive tactics only seemed to get worse as Grace made an effort to understand him better, while Lindsay just began to accept that she couldn't count on Ron and gave up demanding much of anything from him.

Lindsay and Grace began to feel like puppets, with Ron and Harry pulling the strings. If you feel the same way—that you're working hard to communicate and resolve issues and yet your partner seems to be sabotaging these efforts by withholding the effort needed to collaborate and by withdrawing—you too need to establish and reinforce new boundaries (B).

Lindsay's New Boundaries

- **Unacceptable:** When Ron begins to get mad, he often stops talking and minimally or barely answers when I talk to him or ask him questions.

- **Acceptable:** Ron will look at me and pay attention when I speak with him, provided I clearly get his attention at a reasonable time (e.g., not in the middle of his favorite ball game or when he is engrossed in reading). He will talk with me about the issue I've raised until we reach resolution or mutually decide to stop talking.

- **Unacceptable:** When I try to talk with Ron or ask him a question, he will often tell me that I'm nagging him or overreacting and retreat to another part of the house. He often will separate from me for hours at a time until I go to him and plead with him to be with me again.

- **Acceptable:** Ron will remain in the room with me until our issue is resolved to our mutual satisfaction. He will take responsibility for discussing and resolving any issues that arise.

- **Unacceptable:** Ron fails to do his part around the house. He either fails to do those tasks he has agreed to do or does them in a manner that is incomplete and must be finished by me or they won't get done.

- **Acceptable:** Ron will fully complete agreed-on tasks in the agreed-on time frame.

Grace's New Boundaries

Grace decided to focus on one new boundary that seemed to capture what felt most disrespectful and frustrating about Harry's passive expression of anger: his avoidance of verbally committing himself to an opinion or emotion. After much consideration, she worded her boundary as follows:

- **Unacceptable:** When I ask Harry for his opinion or to define how he feels, he refuses to commit himself by saying some version of "I don't care," "I don't know," or "It doesn't matter, anyway," and then ignores me or walks away.

- **Acceptable:** When I ask him his opinion or how he feels (at a reasonable time), he will stop what he is doing, show interest (e.g., look at me, move his facial muscles to show he's listening), and make a good-faith effort to consider and reply. This requires him to avoid any immediate use of the "I don't know or care" litany. After considering my question, he will offer an answer, even if it is to express that he has not made up his mind and needs more time to think about it.

Rearranging Your Thinking to Support Your Acting (C)

Before considering how they would present and reinforce their new boundaries with their partners, Lindsay and Grace needed to identify core beliefs (see the Beliefs Checklist in Chapter 4) that seemed to stand in the way of change. For each unhelpful belief they identified, they crafted a factual and positive counterbelief, shown in the sidebar on the facing page.

Identifying the major stumbling blocks in their old beliefs made both Grace and Lindsay feel they had more personal control than before. Now they had to banish those old beliefs and make the new ones stick. This meant immediately challenging any self-talk that supported the unhelpful beliefs while quickly stating their new belief to themselves. The new boundaries both had drawn also served to strengthen these new beliefs and build more self-confidence.

Self-talk that is not based on observable facts and that incorporates no plan for resolution of a problem is a cognitive distortion, as you know from Chapter 4. Lindsay and Grace examined cognitive distortions like the following. Do any of them sound familiar to you? If so, think about what thoughts you often have about your life with your partner's passive anger and *how those thoughts make you feel*.

"I can't cope with the way he withdraws from me."

Lindsay could see immediately that this thought was not objective but was an example of being *self-deprecating*. This distortion is harmful because it contributes to anxiety and dread about life with a passive–aggressive partner, keeping Lindsay stuck in the automatic pilot mode of reacting to Ron in the same ways and allowing the status quo to persist. Lindsay decided to challenge her "can't cope" self-talk with factual thoughts that included an optimistic aspiration or specific plan:

"[FACT] I control how I act and react, and I can cope if I have a new plan. [PLAN] I will go for a walk to relax myself and then figure out what I wish to do."

"[FACT] Making myself upset only makes my life feel out of control. [PLAN] I need to think about this factually and decide what I can do right now to feel better."

To craft a counterbelief, try starting with the polar opposite of the mistaken idea and embellish it to fit your taste and personal goals.

Grace's Unhelpful Beliefs	Grace's Counterbeliefs
"I am powerless to change the situation I am in."	"I can and will change and will not let Harry's passive anger control me anymore!"
"Nothing seems to work to get him to change. It's hopeless!"	"I have many new ideas and tactics to change myself. I am powerless over Harry but totally powerful over myself."
"Harry can't change due to his past."	"Maybe his past affects how he acts, but I *can* change how I am coping with his passive anger."
"Things will work out if I give it enough time."	"I choose to act *now* to change my life in this relationship."

Lindsay's Unhelpful Beliefs	Lindsay's Counterbeliefs
"I am powerless to change the situation I am in."	"I am powerful over my situation and can change myself, which will make things better."
"He will always win in the end."	"This is not about winning or losing; it's about sticking to my boundaries and making my life better."
"It's my fault when Ron gets angry. I've asked for too much."	"Ron controls his anger. I will make reasonable requests and am powerless over how he feels and acts."
"I am too stressed out and overwhelmed to cope. I don't feel strong enough to deal with him most of the time."	"Ron's actions are what stress me most, and I am taking steps to cope in a way that will bring me more peace and control. I *can* do this."
"Everyone has problems like ours. I shouldn't complain."	"What 'everyone' has is not the issue. I am changing to make *my* life better!"

"[FACT] I have options for myself even if Ron doesn't choice to change. [PLAN] For example, I can go to the movies myself, call a friend to go out for dinner, or download a good movie. If Ron doesn't want to participate, it is his choice and loss."

The more Lindsay focused on the actual facts about her own strengths and choices and opened her awareness to new behaviors she could use to cope (a plan), the less she focused on Ron and her "plight." Her rebuttals may seem pretty basic affirmations of reality, but compared to her negative self-talk they really helped her feel more empowered and focused on what she could do without waiting for Ron to change.

How would this kind of thinking, which Grace discovered in her Daily Log, make you feel?

"I feel he is running this relationship with his passive ways. He always gets what he wants in the end because I can't stand feeling so alone."

Grace concluded there was a lot of sad truth in this one. She acknowledged that Harry's negative actions were "running" her emotions and thus ruling her actions. However, she also began to see that this was a choice on her part—not a permanent fact. Moreover, he usually did get what he wanted, she saw, because of her fears. When asked what her core fear about Harry was, Grace answered, "I guess I get so upset because I thought we would always be together, and now I can't stand the way we relate to each other. Maybe I'm afraid I will just have enough and leave and then be alone. The idea of being on my own and dating again is really upsetting to think about. I guess I just put up with a lot so I don't have to deal with my real feelings. I'm unhappy and afraid to do anything about it."

Grace's daily apprehension that Harry would withdraw from her became much more understandable when she uncovered what she was truly trying to avoid. Her strong need to be loved and cared for in a safe, predictable environment were being blocked by Harry's inconsistent and arbitrary approach to reassuring her. He was so up and down in his communication and intimate behavior with her that she was constantly feeling threatened at a deeper level: "Will he be here for me when I need him? Will this relationship continue?" Grace decided to recast this unhelpful set of thoughts and to replace them with positive affirma-tions that were based on fact, like this one:

"[FACT] I run my own life and can decide what I need from Harry and what is unacceptable. He decides what he does about that, but either way, I run my own life. [PLAN] I will focus on getting fit and healthy and finding other activities to do when Harry refuses to participate or shuts me out."

Lindsay and Grace wrote their new beliefs and some supportive ideas for self-talk on an index card to be kept close by where they could read it every day, whenever unhelpful self-talk cropped up. They also used their Daily Logs to vent feelings of anxiety, worry, guilt, or anger, to remind them of how their thinking impacts their emotions, and to keep track of their progress. A key to success with cognitive-behavioral programs like the one in the A–E model is to keep working on the changes in your thoughts. Lindsay worked every day on catching her old thoughts and actions and trying to immediately challenge them. Sometimes she was more successful than others. Sometimes Ron would still get to her, but she soon began to notice that his passive–aggression was losing its sting and she could recover and move on more quickly. Besides, by thinking more positively and confidently she began to feel better about herself—regardless of what Ron did or didn't do! This alone felt like a victory.

As you now know, however, just altering your thinking isn't enough. How would Lindsay react to Ron's passive anger from now on? How could Grace uphold her new beliefs that she was in control of herself and could decide what was acceptable treatment from Harry and what wasn't? How could they both communicate effectively and reinforce their new bound-aries with their partners in a way that would defuse conflict and foster

Don't discard your Daily Log once you've recorded your reactions to your partner's anger for a couple of weeks. Continue to make entries for as long as your partner's anger is a problem for you. Looking back over it can be a great source of enlightenment and encouragement (e.g., you can compare how you once thought and felt to how you are currently handling things better). You can also quickly identify when you are beginning to have a setback (e.g., your old thinking and actions are rearing their heads again) and use the tools in Chapter 10 to get back on track.

better communication in the long run? In simple words, both Grace and Lindsay needed a new plan.

Putting Your Plan into Action (D and E)

Lindsay and Grace had the same concerns about how to express their expectations and deny their partners any rewards for passive anger that you probably have: How do you find the right time and situation to begin to communicate your new boundaries while not setting off World War III or a new Cold War? When your partner continues his or her passive ways, how do you sustain your resolve not to reward this dysfunctional behavior in any way while maintaining your own self-esteem and position?

Rehearsals: At my request, Lindsay and Grace identified scenarios they thought were likely when they confronted their partners with their passive anger. Each crafted a set of new responses that would support her boundaries and assert her position and then practiced with me or a close friend or in her imagination until she felt she got it right (see Chapter 5 on rehearsals). Here are three examples that will help you emerge with a template for your own new strategy with your partner.

Lindsay: Practicing How to Respond When Ron Makes Excuses

Ron fails to follow through with a task he has agreed to do yet clearly resents. When confronted, he often complains that he is under too much stress at work to find the energy to get things done. In this scenario Lindsay uses an "I" message to restate her boundary that Ron take responsibility for tasks he agreed to do and to confront his excuses.

> LINDSAY: Ron, I see that you didn't clean up the kitchen as you agreed to since I was working late [unacceptable behavior]. As you know, I expect you to follow through with what you agree to do, with no excuses [acceptable alternative action]. I feel really disappointed and confused and would ask you to do it now.
>
> RON: (*Sighs and turns away to read his newspaper.*) I am sorry. I was so exhausted when I got in I just didn't get to it. I'll do it later.
>
> LINDSAY: I expect you to follow through. We are both stressed and tired. If you don't, I will fix dinner for myself and you can fix

your own. I will not keep reminding you to follow through or nag any longer. I will just move forward with my own life, and you can either participate as a partner or fend for yourself.

RON: What is this, tit for tat? Why can't you care about me and my feelings?

LINDSAY: This is about what I am willing to do and not do. I will no longer remind you of your obligations. If you can't or won't do your part, I am moving on to get things done in whatever way works for me.

Everything Lindsay does—using an "I" message, speaking calmly and politely, being behaviorally specific, and not getting hooked into his excuses or pleadings—puts Lindsay in control of herself. She invites Ron to uphold his agreements and sets the stage to move on with her life if he doesn't. She is no longer a captive of what he doesn't do.

Grace: Practicing How to Respond When Harry Won't Commit

Grace wants Harry to commit himself to plans for the upcoming summer. Yet it feels like the more she has reminded him that they need to talk and plan, the more he withholds any commitment to discuss the issues. She confronts him using her newfound tools.

GRACE: Harry, I have asked you now at least three times to sit down and decide on some vacation plans so we can begin to book flights and hotels. I feel frustrated that each time I bring this up you put me off, and you've just done it again [unacceptable behavior]. This is unacceptable to me, and I need you to talk with me in a direct, clear manner this weekend, or I will decide myself and book our plans [acceptable alternative action]. If you don't like what I plan, it is on you. I will be happy. Your satisfaction with the summer is up to you.

HARRY: You wouldn't do that behind my back, would you? You need to discuss this with me at a better time.

GRACE: I have already tried to get you to discuss this on multiple occasions. I am frustrated and finished. Unless you tell me what your ideas are by this weekend, I will commit us financially to plans for a holiday of my choosing. I will no longer be stuck by

your unwillingness to participate in decisions and then complaining. If you don't like the holiday I set up, don't come. I will
go with my cousin. Let me know what you decide.

Notice that Grace does not let herself become trapped in Harry's
withholding behavior. She sets her boundary: she expects him to participate and, if not, clearly states her intended actions, which are no longer
based on what he does or fails to do. His outcome is created by his own
action or inaction (logical and natural consequence), and Grace is free of
his passive–aggressive control over her life.

Grace: Practicing How to Respond When Harry Won't Open Up about His Feelings

Not only does Harry fail to commit himself to decisions as a passive tactic, he also is unwilling to discuss his thoughts and feelings with Grace.
She has often questioned him to a point of frustration and spends much
time "having to be a mind reader," a job she didn't apply for and hates.
Grace tries to apply as many of the "guidelines" as she can as she assertively confronts Harry:

> GRACE: Harry, you just made a face when I told you my mother is
> coming over. What are you feeling? Do you want her to come?
>
> HARRY: (*Rolls his eyes and sighs loudly.*) What are you talking about?
> If she's coming, she's coming. I don't really care.
>
> GRACE: I've asked you nicely, and you refuse to commit yourself or
> tell me how you feel about it [unacceptable behavior]. I won't
> continue to ask. Unless you tell me clearly and directly how
> you feel about it [acceptable alternative action], she will arrive
> at noon for lunch.
>
> HARRY: (*raising his voice*) I can't believe how you talk to me. I am not
> a child! I just know she'll come no matter what I say. You are
> in control.
>
> GRACE: (*using the "broken record" from Chapter 5*) As I said, when you
> are ready to tell me how you feel in a clear, direct way, I will
> listen and try to work with you. (*Leaves the room.*)

Notice in this scenario how Harry tries to redirect the discussion
toward how Grace treats him, still avoiding answering her original reasonable question. Instead of getting sucked into defending herself, which

was her old pattern, she now merely restates her request for acceptable behavior using the "broken record" strategy of calmly repeating her request. She stays on point and will no longer permit herself to be derailed by his avoidance tactics. Grace can now feel free to enjoy her day with her mother, and Harry can either participate or not. It is his only choice. Disrupting the day or "punishing" Grace with his passive anger is no longer an option.

The Importance of Praising Acceptable Behavior

Incidentally, it's important to let your passive–aggressive or coldly angry partner know, in behaviorally specific language, when his or her actions are acceptable and welcome. The "I" message is just as effective for praising as for giving negative feedback. If this sounds as if you'll be treating your partner like a child, remember that using positive feedback or praise is a powerful way of encouraging new behavior for all of us. Here are some examples of affirming "I" messages:

> GRACE: Harry, you just answered me immediately when I asked you about your day at work. When you acknowledge me like that, I feel you really appreciate me, which makes me happy. I really appreciate your making this kind of effort. Thanks.

> LINDSAY: Ron, thanks for remembering to pick up the groceries on your way home. Following through on something I asked you to do makes me feel really cared for. It's incredibly reassuring. Thanks!

> GRACE: You just told me exactly how you feel. I'm listening, and I'm really pleased that you told me this. I want you to know I'll take your feelings about this into account. How do you think we should proceed [to resolve this issue]?

You probably noticed the leap we just made from your changing *your* act to your expressing gratitude for your partner's changing *his* act. Obviously, the assumption is that the changes you make will encourage your partner to make the changes you seek. I hope that does indeed happen for you. But there are plenty of times when it won't. And there will be times when change will be a challenge for you too, because old beliefs and actions are well learned and can be replaced with new ones only with significant practice. Expect to encounter setbacks and obstacles along the way. Chapter 10 helps prepare you for these possibilities and offers some solutions you can try when you encounter pitfalls.

PART III

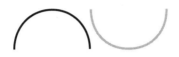

Making
Boundaries Stick

10

COPING
WITH THE EXPECTED
AND PREPARING
FOR THE UNKNOWN

You now have a wide repertoire of strategies for dealing with your partner's anger. Maybe you've already seen how using them can change the outcome of heated interactions and icy standoffs. New responses from you can be surprisingly powerful on their own. With time and persistence, they might transform your entire relationship.

But they come with no guarantees. You're bound to encounter resistance from your partner. And at times you might resent having to do all the work and find yourself slipping back into old anger routines that allow your partner to pick up where he or she left off. Being ready for typical obstacles and knowing how to regroup when progress halts will get you back on track.

DEALING WITH RESISTANCE
FROM YOUR PARTNER

Once you start using the strategies in this book, your partner can no longer act out stress, pent-up anger, or grievances in any way that is unacceptable to you and expect you to tolerate it. But will your partner see the error of his or her ways and start to change along with you? Probably not at first. Many people like your partner end up left behind to stew in the juices of ineffectual anger expression. This may seem like a sad outcome—it's certainly not the best-case scenario you would have preferred—but that stewing is often necessary for real change to occur in the future.

Whether or not—and when—your partner changes will depend on his or her degree of stubbornness, the strength of old habits, and even the existence of underlying serious mental illness or traits. In my experience people with anger issues rarely change overnight because managing anger requires:

- A lot of personal motivation

- A thorough understanding of underlying beliefs

- Identification of what triggers anger

- Tools to dampen anger arousal quickly before the flame of anger gets out of control

If your partner seems open to change at all, you might offer him or her my previous book, *Taking Charge of Anger* or refer to my website (see Suggested Resources), which is designed to help your partner (or you) to express anger in appropriate and acceptable ways. Having such tools at his disposal may be just what your partner needs to get over the hump and on the road to personal change. Meanwhile, however, you need to stay the course. While your partner stews, his brain is absorbing the idea that your boundaries remain firm and he's not getting what his anger used to provide. Change might eventually start to seem worth considering.

Why Is This So Hard?

Can you relate to any of these thoughts and feelings?

"No matter what I say, he seems to have an answer and won't admit he needs to change, let alone get some help with his anger."

"I'm feeling overwhelmed with trying to stand up for myself. It just isn't working."

Change Is Hard ...
But Not Impossible

If necessity is the mother of invention, then lack of necessity is the mother of inertia. No one wants to invest energy into changing when things seem just fine as they are. Ever stayed in a home long after your family had outgrown it? Eaten the same tired menu over and over even though you craved something new? Keep these tendencies in mind when your partner seems unwilling to get with the new anger-expression program and you're about ready to throw in the towel. Your partner may not want to change because being able to vent anger with someone who accepts him or her no matter what has felt pretty comfortable—a lot more comfortable than doing the work to bring it under control. Of course you've changed the ground rules now, and if you uphold them, your partner's sense of comfort is probably dwindling more every day.

Also remind yourself that your partner may have come by bad habits in identifying and communicating anger from a number of inner sources:

- Your partner may never have learned to communicate feelings.

- Your partner may have a serious emotional problem like depression or personality disturbance that must be addressed by a professional.

- Your partner may be under a lot of life stress that releases his or her emotions and results in more impulsive acting out.

None of these is an excuse for imposing anger on you. But knowing that factors beyond your partner's control may have shaped his behavior can help you remain empathic and patient while your partner struggles with the urge to resist change that seems so obviously desirable to you.

The good news is that over time we become accustomed to the idea of change the longer we're confronted with it, just like we got so comfortable with the way we did things in the past. (Remember how foreign texting on your phone seemed at first? Do you catch yourself feeling impatient with those who don't check their e-mail constantly?)

"Why does this have to be so difficult? Why doesn't she just get it and stop arguing that she's not to blame? I am not blaming her; I just want peace."

"I seem to get drawn into my old behavior so easily! Why is this so hard?"

Self-help methods like the A–E model you've been learning sound simple so that (1) you can absorb and remember the steps easily and (2) you can quickly call up strategies and solutions in the heat of those moments when you need them most. That doesn't mean the process you undergo will actually be straightforward or simple. Life is not a bowl of cherries, and this is no cookbook. You can't just mix the new responses you've learned and bake up a new life with your partner. Factors much more complex than inferior ingredients or a faulty oven will stand in the way of a perfect result.

Primary among these is that your partner may try to keep things as they are to get you to give up and return to your old ways of accepting behavior that you've now designated unacceptable. Your patience will be tested, and it may begin to seem that setting new boundaries is just too difficult. In fact, it may seem that your partner's anger is getting worse, not better.

The Extinction Burst

Psychologists have long recognized that when old behavior (your partner's old face of anger) is no longer rewarded it begins to extinguish and may eventually disappear altogether. This process is never smooth. It may produce an *extinction burst*, a well-studied phenomenon in which the undesirable behavior begins to occur even more often than before. It is a kind of last-ditch effort of your partner to get you to return to permitting or rewarding his or her anger. Its goal is maintenance of the status quo. An extinction burst may be frightening, as when your partner withdraws for an even longer time or ups the ante with a dramatic meltdown. All this will test your patience and may make setting new boundaries seem in vain. But it is predictable, and you must stay the course of your new behavior even if it seems things are getting worse. (Of course, if your partner becomes violent, you need to take more drastic action; see Chapter 8.)

The Many Faces of Resistance to Change

Once your partner realizes you're no longer dancing to her tune, she'll probably start to pull out all the stops when you try to confront her anger. Each of the following blocking/defending responses is somewhat unique, but mostly they occur in pairs or threesomes (e.g., denial plus blaming and minimizing) as your partner attempts to leave no room for you to continue the confrontation. Fortunately, you have effective options for responding and breaking down your partner's resistance. You've read about many of these types of responses before, but now you are going to read about them again in the context of partner resistance because each of the following roadblocks can be addressed effectively only if you are aware of what they are, when they arise, and what response from you will work best. If not, you may be so caught up in defending yourself or justifying your position that you lose sight of what is actually happening: your partner is trying to derail your new behavior.

"This isn't working! You're only ruining our relationship! You're just wasting time."

Remember Jenny from Chapter 3? James's intense outbursts, particularly when he was drinking, had become very frightening to her. She didn't think he'd harm her physically—he never had—but she'd had enough of his yelling and threatening to leave. She waited for the right time to discuss her new boundaries with him. He reacted by telling her he knew what she was up to:

> JAMES: Jenny, this is ridiculous! I know you think you can threaten me—control how I express my anger. Well, it won't work with me. This is who I am, and you better learn to accept it. This is who you married.

ROADBLOCK: *UNDERMINING*

Saying "This is who I am—I can't change" is a common form of undermining. In reality, your partner is saying "I refuse to make any efforts to change—so live with things the way they are." By making any change seem impossible, your partner may hope you will be so disheartened that you will give up your new boundaries.

SOLUTION: *PERSISTENCE*

Let your partner know that you cannot control what he decides to do but you are crystal clear about what your boundaries are and you will persist in enforcing them no matter what. You can use the "broken record" defusing approach described in Chapter 5: calmly repeat your boundary and response no matter what roadblock your partner erects to undermine your efforts.

WHAT YOU MIGHT SAY:

> JENNY: It may seem that way to you, but I again state that I expect you to use a calm and respectful approach whenever you speak with me. If not, I will immediately stop the discussion until you can calmly discuss your feelings with me [broken record].
>
> JAMES: But that's not fair to me! Why can't you understand how much I go through every day? That's what sets me off.
>
> JENNY: (*One more time Jenny repeats her new boundary—broken record—not getting pulled into a discussion of James's stress or rationalizations for his hostility. After this she walks away.*)

"Everybody gets mad sometimes."

Sean's excuse for his anger with Cara (Chapter 5) was to tell her that he is no different from anyone else: "It's no big deal." Jack told Pamela (Chapter 6) that his scary blowups and hostility to others were not really his fault. "Our problem is that I'm under stress and you can't really understand how hard it is for me every day. Sure, I get a bit irritated at times. Who wouldn't?"

ROADBLOCK: *OVERGENERALIZING*

Jack is in complete denial about his hostility and tries the diversionary tactic of claiming that his stress would make anybody get "irritated." That may be true, but it's hardly the point; Pamela's point is about the way Jack expresses his reaction to that stress.

SOLUTION: *BE SPECIFIC AND PERSONAL*

The only way for Pamela to counter overgeneralization is to take the argument in the other direction, getting as specific about what *Jack* does (forget about what others do!) and as personal (how it impacts her) as possible.

WHAT YOU MIGHT SAY:

> JACK: Don't tell me I have this big anger problem. I don't [denial]! Everybody gets mad at times. Who doesn't [overgeneralizing]? So don't tell me this is a big deal.

> PAMELA: Last evening you came in the door loud, complaining and cursing in front of the kids [specific description about Jack, not everyone else]. I asked you to stop. Then I just walked away. What anyone else does is not my problem. Your actions affect me, and I will no longer tolerate them, as I've told you [personal].

"I am just exhausted [or too sick, hurting, too depressed]."

In Chapter 8 you met Hunter, who was often the object of his wife's verbal raging when her chronic back pain got particularly bad. When Hunter announced his new boundary regarding Charlotte's in-your-face aggression, here's how she reacted:

> CHARLOTTE: It is not fair to tell me you won't talk with me when I get upset. You don't care that I am in awful pain!

ROADBLOCK: *MEDICALIZING*

Your partner could be experiencing a real medical problem: clinical depression, chronic back pain, migraine headaches, or any of an unlimited list of others that cause discomfort or outright pain. In Chapter 5 I reviewed five factors—sleep, stress, sustenance, substances, and sickness—that can greatly influence how intensely aroused you or your partner may become when angry. Clearly "sickness" may affect how irritable we get and how much aggravation we can stand before getting angry. When your partner does have a medical issue, it's important to avoid having critical discussions when the illness is flaring up in some way. After all, you want your discussion of boundaries to occur when you are more likely to be heard, and you would hope your partner would extend the same courtesy to you when you're not feeling up to par.

SOLUTION: *IMMOVABLE BOUNDARIES*

However, there is a difference between being empathic and understanding about a medical problem and enabling your partner to use it as an excuse to act out anger in insulting or scary ways. *Draw a line at your new boundary no matter how your partner is feeling.* He or she deserves your care and concern, but you are not signing on to be a doormat or punching bag for your partner's irritation or pain. Here's how Hunter (Chapter 8) dealt with in-your-face aggression from Charlotte, who suffered chronic back pain that often made her irritable, after he had declared his new boundary around her verbal raging.

WHAT YOU MIGHT SAY:

> HUNTER: I do care and will listen to you and try to help when you aren't feeling well. That does not mean I will put up with you yelling in my face or breaking things when you get mad. Use your calm words to tell me how you feel or I won't be present to listen. I will no longer tolerate your using your back pain as an excuse to be mean and insulting to me.

Hunter follows through in this manner anytime Charlotte is verbally aggressive with him.

"I am overwhelmed and too stressed out to worry about getting too loud."

Josh (Chapter 3) found himself increasingly frustrated and hurt by Kathy's dumping job stress on him and their teenage children. Kathy would often arrive home bristling with anger and frustration from her day as a partner in a prestigious law firm. She would rail about clients and partners who failed to meet her high standards. When Josh asked her to talk calmly and not to curse so much in front of the kids, she criticized him with sarcasm and loud insults. He spent much of his life trying to keep stress low at home to avoid setting her off.

ROADBLOCK: *THE STRESS EXCUSE*

This is perhaps the most common justification used to explain away inappropriate expressions of anger. In our busy, changing culture most of us can relate to working hard and being tense or tired at the end of the day. This is no excuse to dump our frustrations on our partners just because we can. Notice I said "can." Our partners love and care for us, and dumping our frustrations and angst on them can become a bad habit. After all, no one else will tolerate our anger for long. This is a sad fact of intimate relationships, also captured in an old song title: "You Always Hurt the One You Love." The fact that most of us can relate to this lamentable behavior doesn't make it right. In some cases, like many cited in this book, the anger that gets dumped is toxic and even abusive.

SOLUTION: *IMMOVABLE BOUNDARIES*

If you are on the receiving end of stress-induced anger, treat it like any unwanted behavior: set your boundary and hold to it no matter what justification your partner proposes. You are willing to talk only if treated with respect ("acceptable" boundary behavior).

Josh had had enough by the time we first spoke. We devised a plan to set a clear boundary for Kathy using the tools found in this book.

WHAT YOU MIGHT SAY:

KATHY: (*loud voice*) I don't want to hear what you need from me. I do enough already around here, earning most of the money to keep this home going. I am stressed out enough without having to deal with your feelings too. Give me a break!

JOSH: I have already given you too many breaks. I know your work is stressful. So is mine. This excuse will no longer work for me. If you are loud and rude, I will call it to your attention one time. If it continues, I will stop talking with you. Period! You can decide how to deal with your stress without using me as a receptacle for your frustrations.

KATHY: (*louder*) Don't you dare try to threaten me. You will listen to me. I earn the right.

JOSH: (*Calmly walks away.*) When you can treat me with calm respect, I will talk with you.

KATHY: Come back here! You coward!

JOSH: (*Goes about his business. When Kathy later calms down and speaks with him in a calm, friendly voice, he immediately resumes talking with her.*)

"I am just no good at that touchy-feely stuff. I am not as
good as you with feelings."

This excuse is used mostly by men, and there's some truth to the claim that men are less skilled at communicating feelings than women. Studies of boys' development by Dr. William Pollack reveal what has been called the "Boy Code," a set of implicit and explicit rules boys are taught by the time they are five or six years old about what kinds of behavior are acceptable. Suffice it to say that talking about feelings like embarrassment, fear, or sadness is not okay among other boys, who might shame the speaker or ignore any "feeling" remarks by changing the subject. Boys learn early on that anger is a very acceptable emotion and most others are not. Girls, on the other hand, begin talking about and expressing feelings early on to determine how they really feel and to establish bonds of friendship via self-disclosure.

ROADBLOCK: *THE INCOMPETENCE EXCUSE*

Dr. Deborah Tannen, a linguist who has studied how men and women communicate, believes that these differences in socialization and learning are responsible for many miscommunications between men and women in intimate relationships. If you don't believe this, just think back to how often you've overheard men describing how "sad and perplexed" they were or how "humiliated and embarrassed" they felt in front of another guy. It almost never happens, as men tend to talk about things and events while women are much more comfortable discussing their feelings with one another.

This discomfort with "feelings talk" is why many men are uncomfortable with the idea of going to counseling. I believe that counselors must make a focused effort to make male clients comfortable and accepted even though they may not be as good as their female counterparts at describing and relating emotionally charged situations.

SOLUTION: *PATIENT UNDERSTANDING AND LISTENING—*
ON BOTH SIDES

This is a tough one. On the one hand, the "I'm not good with feelings" rationalization is not an acceptable excuse for men to act out anger in hurtful ways. On the other hand, there is some truth to the rationalization, meaning that you may have to make efforts when your partner's anger is *not* at a peak to listen carefully and try to understand the feelings that your partner may be having but not understanding fully. Always choose patient understanding in favor of using your prowess to confuse or gain power. For example, avoid saying things like "You never know what you feel, do you!?" or "Why can't you just admit that you're scared?" But when your partner produces the incompetence excuse, you have a right to say calmly that he should do you the courtesy of sitting down across from you and listening with all his attention. If he cannot (or will not) and continues to express anger in ways you've declared unacceptable, follow through with the consequences you've established along with your new boundaries. And then the two of you, with care and good efforts at listening to each other, can work at crossing the divide between men and women on a more regular basis. I suggest you review page 101 in Chapter 5, which shows the verbal and nonverbal components of "Active Listening." Listening in a positive and acknowledging way greatly encourages your partner to express himself. Also, look for resources on communication at the back of this book.

"If you would just go with the flow and be more understanding, we wouldn't be having these problems!"

NED: (to Julie, Chapter 2) The house is too messy and out of control. You don't have any idea how to deal with the kids. Who wouldn't get mad?

JAMES: (to Jenny, Chapter 3) This place is a zoo. What do you do all day? You're teaching our kids to be slobs like you! I've had a miserable day, and I come home to this mess! Of course I'm upset! I'm out of here. (*Walks to the door.*)

JACK: (to Pamela, Chapter 6) It's not my fault I'm ticked off! That stupid car never gets me where I need to go, and I missed a really important meeting today!

POSSIBLY-YOUR-PARTNER: You've known how I am for all these months/years. What's the big deal now?

SAM: (to Lacey, Chapter 8) I'm not the one with the problem—it's your insecurity and lack of empathy and understanding that's the real problem.

ROADBLOCK: *BLAMING*

Blame offers a veritable cornucopia of excuses and deflections to an angry and change-resistant individual. In this all-too-common defensive maneuver your partner blames the messenger for the message, with the goal of removing the focus from your partner, who thinks he or she is being falsely accused. As exemplified by the preceding quotes, blame laying takes several different forms:

Blame Shifting

Here your partner points out that it is your personal deficit that is causing the anger in the first place. This is the blaming tactic favored by both Ned and James.

Other people shift the blame not to you but to just about anything except themselves. This was Jack's typical response to Pamela's statements about his anger. He would blame:

- **Others** who failed to meet his expectations: the baby-sitter who left crumbs on the counter, the cabdriver who took a route Jack didn't agree with, and coworkers who didn't do things Jack's way.

- **Objects** that didn't work as Jack thought they should: for example, Jack couldn't assemble a bicycle and blamed the "incompetent" bike designer; his "stupid" car let him down so he missed a meeting, so he threw a tantrum.

- **Situations** that didn't turn out as expected, like a traffic jam caused by "rude," "lousy," and "incompetent" drivers; thunderstorms that interrupted plane travel; and kids who delayed getting ready on time.

Minimizing

In this form of leveling blame, your partner makes light of your concerns about his or her anger to put you at fault: the problem is supposedly your oversensitivity or tendency to magnify things. Your partner might ask: "What's the big deal? So I get a little mad once in a while."

Psychologizing

Your partner blames his or her anger levels on your emotional problems or deficits. Sam (Chapter 8) blamed his "need" to hold on to Lacey and block her from leaving him on her lack of empathy for his needs and issues. He would stand in front of her and hold on to her arms to keep her from leaving until she would agree to "listen" to him. He justified this by blaming her for not being able to handle problems—for not being able to love him enough to stay with him no matter what. In simple words Sam justified anything he did to keep Lacey a captive to his needs because she was emotionally defective and *he* had to *make her* see the light.

> SAM: If you had just listened to me and stopped talking, this [the abuse] wouldn't have happened.

> SAM: You're just overreacting again. Get over it.

SOLUTION: *IMMOVABLE BOUNDARIES*

You will not be distracted by attempts to blame you. The issue you have raised is your partner's actions and their impact on you. If necessary, use the "broken record" to continue to reiterate your boundaries: "Well, that may be true, but right now I am asking you to [restate boundaries]." Whatever you do, be unwilling to shift the discussion to a critique of you or your behavior. You have opened a discussion about your partner's anger behaviors and will not defend yourself or let the conversation be redirected to your "faults." Here are some tactics that Julie and Jenny used with their partners to make their boundaries immovable.

> JULIE: (to Ned) Whether or not you think the house is messy is not the point. Losing your cool and yelling and berating me must stop, or I will not be available to talk. If you talk with me in a calm and friendly manner, I will be happy to discuss any issue you have.

> JENNY: (to James) When James tries to deflect the conversation away from his behavior and to "the house is a zoo," Jenny uses the same approach as Julie: reiterating that she will not be moved from her enforcement of her new boundaries. When he persists in criticizing her in a mean and cutting tone of voice, calling her "out of her mind," she calmly leaves the situation and uses the "STOP" strategy discussed in Chapter 5.

"I will not discuss my anger again. It's your problem, so get over it!"

Refusing to talk about an issue has been reviewed before in this book. It is a powerful nonverbal tactic to derail resolution of a topic and often a way to punish you by not giving you what you want (a form of cold anger).

ROADBLOCK: *STONEWALLING*

As noted earlier, John Gottman has studied what makes relationships succeed or fail by carefully observing videotapes of couples' interactions. Stonewalling is one of what he calls the "Four Horsemen" of negative behaviors that predict serious problems in a relationship (the others are criticizing, defensiveness, and contempt). Stonewalling usually takes one of two forms:

Denial

Your partner maintains there is no problem. You are wrong, and he or she is just not doing the things you are alleging. This is often the case with versions of passive anger. You may recall Vince and Melissa from Chapter 7. Melissa refused to acknowledge that she was angry with Vince following occasions when she would put him down with sarcasm or tell personal stories or jokes at his expense. For example, his Daily Log showed her saying things like:

> "Vince, what are you talking about? I was only pulling your leg. Get a life!"

> "Vince, you are totally too sensitive! No one seemed to care about your job [after she told their friends that Vince was passed over for promotion without getting his permission to discuss this embarrassing topic], and you are overreacting as usual. And I am not trying to hurt you. Ever!"

SOLUTION: *STRESS PERSONAL IMPACT*

If your partner decides to stonewall you when you try to discuss new boundaries, all you can do is to state your boundaries clearly even if he or she refuses to have a mutual discussion. The best response to denial in particular is to focus on your personal reaction or impact and to refuse to debate whether the person did something or meant to do something to hurt you in some fashion. Your own impact cannot be disputed (it is *your* inner set of feelings and thoughts) even if your partner claims no intent to harm you. Review these responses to statements that deny negative intent:

> MELISSA: Vince, I didn't mean to embarrass you in any way. I would never hurt you."
>
> VINCE: (*focusing on his personal impact*) That may be so, Melissa, but when you told our friends that I was passed over at work, I **felt humiliated and embarrassed—no matter what you intended**. In the future, please do not tell anything personal about me unless you clear it with me first.

Recall David's sarcastic comments to Angela (Chapter 7) about her taste and efforts to remodel their home. Angela took offense and told him so. David denies a negative intent.

> DAVID: I don't mean to put you down. When I said something about your ideas for the house, it wasn't to hurt you but to help make things better. I care about you.
>
> ANGELA: No matter what you meant, in my opinion you have demeaned my taste and judgment about making our home more presentable, have mocked my ideas, and put me down to my face or in front of the kids. You don't just offer a suggestion; I feel put down as a person. Your put-downs make me feel worthless, embarrass me, and hurt unbelievably. I will not tolerate your hurtful words any longer.

Cold Withdrawal

Your partner leaves or refuses to talk further when you confront his or her anger. This is the most basic form of cold anger. You may have experienced being frozen out by friends as a kid and know how it can hurt when someone you care about avoids you or won't talk. It's even worse if you are told "No, there's nothing wrong!" when you know something is the matter. In this primitive form of denial, your partner just refuses to talk, either about the subject of his or her anger or about anything you bring up, to punish you. Either way, this is a regressive, infantile way of acting, and you should make it clear right away that you will not make any attempt at begging or cajoling your partner into talking. It is his or her right to act this way, but you are disappointed by such antics.

Jared's approach to managing Greta's cold anger (Chapter 2) was ineffective. Greta would avoid talking to Jared for days at a time when she was mad at him. He would mostly give in and tell her what she wanted to hear as a way of getting her to be with him again. Yet he often felt "hurt, humiliated, and wimpy" when he allowed himself to be seduced into placating her, and this behavior continued unabated whenever she was upset with him. Here are his new boundaries:

• **Unacceptable:** Any form of withdrawal or refusal to talk or interact with him. He told her he would not pursue her and would go on with his life until she decided to approach him again.

• **Acceptable:** She would tell him directly and clearly what she thought and felt. He agreed to listen to her feelings and try to understand them as best he could, whether he agreed with them or not.

When he asked Greta to hear his new boundaries (he selected a time when they were not in conflict), she told Jared she did not want to discuss this issue. His feelings were his "problem." When he persisted in a polite tone of voice, she got up and went to their bedroom, telling him he had again caused the problems between them.

SOLUTION: *BROKEN RECORD*

> JARED: I am sad that you see me as the problem. I want to discuss new ways of handling differences, but you clearly are not ready for that. When you decide to talk with me about these issues, I will make time. Until then, I will not disturb you and will go on with my afternoon.

Unlike in the past, he did not go into the bedroom or entreat Greta to talk to him. By the next day she approached him as if nothing was wrong, and he again stated his desire to have a talk, which they eventually did. He stayed the course, calmly repeating his request using the "broken record" strategy from Chapter 5.

"I am starting to hate you when you go on and on."

Some people quickly resort to emotional blackmail when confronted about their anger. Or they let you know that if you continue to confront them, something you value on a visceral level will be at risk: you might lose their love, your financial stability, your marriage, or even your physical safety and well-being.

ROADBLOCK: *THREATS*

Threats to your life status (your relationship, your finances, the love you count on from your partner), or threats to embarrass you or to hurt you in some way, emotionally or physically, are a way to try to get you to back off. Threats generally come in two varieties: threats to love and security and threats to safety.

Threats to Love and Security

Your partner leads you to believe that if you persist in your new boundaries you are somehow destroying his or her love for you:

> "You are killing my love for you when you won't talk to me [e.g., when you cut off a nasty conversation]."

> "I am fed up and can't take your constant nagging any longer!"

Your partner may even imply or state that he or she may leave you if you persist in enforcing your boundaries. Threats to spend more time with friends (out of the house), to go on a trip alone, or to separate are among the possible tactics. How about these gems:

> "If things don't change, I'm out of here!"

> "I will take the kids and go as far away as I can if you don't [do what I want]."

> "Why do I put up with your garbage? In 24 hours I can find a woman who will treat me better than you!"

SOLUTION: *IMMOVABLE BOUNDARIES*

Interpret such threats for what they are: blackmail. Blackmail is so insidious that we have strict laws against it in our penal code. Blackmail in intimate relationships is harder to prove but easy to identify when you're the target. No matter what, do not give in to it. If you receive any form of threat from your partner, who is trying to get you to continue to put up with his or her anger, your only rational response is to stay the course with your boundaries NO MATTER WHAT IS THREATENED. Let your partner know you will not be intimidated by any form of threat and will not budge in any way from expecting acceptable—reasonable, civilized, and respectful—behavior. What do you think of an approach like this one, which fully upholds your position?

> YOUR PARTNER: You are ruining our relationship with all this talk of your boundaries. I can't be with someone who is so rigid about me expressing my feelings [threat]. So I get angry some-times. I can't help it [denial]. Don't make such a big deal of it [minimizing] if you want me around [threat].

> YOU: I am sad you see me standing up for myself as "ruining" our relationship. Your threatening to leave and minimizing my feelings won't work. I expect you to handle your anger in the acceptable way I outlined from now on. I won't be a part of any more hostility or threats from you.

If your partner can't love you for the confident and assertive person you are trying to become, a person who will not succumb to intimidation or threats, then so be it. Why would you want to stay with someone who cannot accept that you want to live a life without threats and conditional love (e.g., "I will love you only if you do what I want!")? If you have trou-ble asserting these rights, you need the support of a counselor who can help you get strong enough to set firm boundaries and hold to them.

Threats to Safety

I suggest you carefully review Chapter 8 if your partner is in any form or fashion threatening your safety or that of your loved ones.

SOLUTION: LEAVE

Any threat to your safety should be taken seriously, and you should leave or call for help if necessary to find a safe place to stay. Also

access the kinds of resources found in the Suggested Resources section at the end of the book.

Using Enlightened Self-Interest to Get around Roadblocks

Previously, I encouraged readers to exercise a measure of empathy about their partners' lack of emotional skills (without excusing anger in the name of that deficit). But empathy can be a dangerous trap when you're trying to protect your new anger boundaries.

Remember to keep in the forefront of your mind your *own needs* for more peace and quality in this relationship. If you yield to pressure to focus on your partner's discomfort or needs too much, your own will recede to the background where they languished in the past.

Perhaps that's why you wanted to change things in the first place: you've been spending so much time focused on helping your partner with his or her anger/frustrations that you haven't focused on your own needs at all. Now is the time to help yourself. Use the ideas I've just presented to ward off any detours away from your new boundaries. This is not selfish, but enlightened self-interest!

SETBACKS: A GUIDE TO GET YOU BACK ON TRACK

As I said at the beginning of this chapter, erecting and protecting new boundaries is not easy. Along the way you may find that you let down your guard and slip back into old behavior.

After working with the A–E model for about one month, Jenny (Chapter 3) felt she was "back to base one" with James. Again she found herself succumbing to James's accusations that she was selfish and cold when she refused to listen to him when his temper flared.

> JAMES: If you really cared about *me* and not yourself, you would try to understand that I don't mean to get so angry. It just happens when I get stressed out. Please don't let us down and pull away from me. [roadblocks: stress, blaming]

> JAMES: If you were more affectionate and a better wife, I could be

more loving to you. I wouldn't get so mad. [roadblock: blaming]

When I asked Jenny how she felt when he accused her, she told me the guilt was overwhelming and she found herself back to rationalizing, apologizing (see Chapter 2), and giving in to his requests and demands. This was an old, well-worn script between them and a pattern often seen by professionals who work with relationship abuse.

If you find yourself feeling anxious, sad, angry, or guilty in ways that remind you of the past, review the table "Core Emotions, Goals, and Unhelpful Reactions in Response to Your Partner's Anger" in Chapter 2. Uncomfortable emotions like guilt and anxiety arise naturally when you push the envelope a bit in asserting yourself while your partner's energy to roadblock you seems boundless. But if you let those emotions persist, they will only intensify, leading very quickly to old behaviors like editing, rationalizing, justifying, and surrendering. Be aware that this sequence of emotions and actions can happen without much consciousness on your part unless you are prepared to recognize it. If you feel like "all of a sudden" you are back to your old habits and don't quite know how you got there, you'll benefit considerably from the strategies that follow.

Was Jenny really back to base one? When you have a setback, it can certainly feel that way. You are starting to feel and act like you once did. Your old thinking rears its head, and you wonder if you are really accomplishing anything. Your partner may collude in your doubts by trying to

---

Getting Dragged Back into an Old Pattern of Abuse

Can you relate to this sequence of events that Jenny experienced over and over?

1. James would lose his temper and rail at Jenny.
2. He would apologize but blame his anger on her or stress.
3. She would feel guilty and forgive him. ("After all, he doesn't mean to yell and say those things—he's a good man.")
4. He would soon get angry again, followed by another outburst.
5. He would again rationalize and apologize.

undermine your efforts: "Why do you keep trying to start these fights? Just let me work on this and I will change. Trust me."

I said "when" you have a setback, because setbacks are a part of how we learn any new set of behaviors. We begin by trying out new thinking and actions, and through practice (repetition and rehearsal) they start to become automatic and comfortable. Gradually our old habits weaken. But this change takes time, and when we are distracted, stressed, or otherwise vulnerable our old habits will sometimes win out. Setbacks shouldn't convince you to give up your journey; you'll only end up sitting by the side of the road feeling defeated and despairing. Think of a setback as a detour and not a destination.

WHY YOU MIGHT EXPERIENCE A SETBACK

When you know what might cause a setback, you're better prepared to prevent setbacks and to devise a plan to get back on course should one occur.

Not Enough Practice

The most likely reason for your setback in implementing these new ideas is you just haven't learned new thinking and actions to a point where they are automatic. Learning any new skill takes time and practice. Doing multiplication, shooting a basket or passing a football, and driving a car all had one thing in common: to learn them you had to repeat the new behavior again and again. These rehearsals eventually led to your being able to master new behaviors to a point where they became automatic. You could depend on doing well without much thinking or preparation: they became well learned.

The same process must occur in learning to assert your new boundaries. The more you practice standing up for yourself and coping with whatever roadblock your partner throws up, the more your new behavior will occur without much thinking. It will be so well learned that it cannot be derailed easily. In turn, your old reactions to your partner will begin to fall away from disuse. Since they are no longer rehearsed, they are soon placed further back in your memory. Importantly, they are not gone but in "cold storage," as if in a locker in the basement of your mind. You must stay on course to reinforce your new habits and to keep the old ones in deep storage.

In addition to using your new behaviors directly with your partner as anger arises, you can practice with imaginal rehearsals as I first described in Chapter 5.

Practicing in Your Mind When Your Partner Is Not Around

Pick out difficult situations you might face with your partner (Jenny, for example, could imaginally practice how she will respond to James when he throws blame in her direction). Here are the steps I recommend for a good imaginal workout.

- **Close your eyes and vividly picture** a scenario that seems particularly difficult to cope with. Take a few minutes to set the stage: where you are, who is present, what you are both doing. Once you have captured the setting, vividly picture what your partner is doing or saying. Perhaps she is saying something contemptuous to you when angry about a situation that didn't go well. Hear what she is saying and her tone of voice. See her face and body expression as she is saying something that feels mean and insulting.

- **Let yourself feel** as you might naturally feel when she does this. Remember that imagery, if realistic, often provokes the same emotion as the real-life situation (recall how emotional you can get when dreaming or lying awake at night, picturing something bad that happened that day). Images are read by your brain in a way similar to the real-life situation.

- **Now open your eyes and think about your options.** When this situation arises the next time, how can you think about it objectively and optimistically (see Chapter 4) to elicit confidence and calm determination? What positive belief and self-talk will best help you address your partner's challenging actions? Now consider how you can best assert your position in a way that does not reward your partner's actions and clearly states your boundary.

- Finally, close your eyes and let yourself get back into the "action" of your imagination. **Imagine the same challenging situation, except this time imagine you are using your new thoughts and actions to stand up to your partner.** If it feels powerful and effective to you, rehearse it again in imagination until it feels natural and automatic.

You are now prepared to cope with this challenging situation if your partner throws it at you. You will feel more confident and have these new behaviors at the ready in your mind to guide your actions.

Regression

Have you ever witnessed a thirty-year-old man have a meltdown when his kids or the traffic finally got to him? As he is screaming and crying out in anger and frustration, it kind of reminds you of how a three-year-old solves his frustrations, doesn't it? We all have the past learnings and experiences of each age of our development locked into our memory banks. For some reason, when we are really stressed and threatened, we seem to retrieve old and familiar behaviors, drawn from the cold storage of our memories as I discussed earlier. Unhelpful habits of the past, like walking on eggshells around our partners or editing and redirecting what we say and do to keep the peace, may rear their heads just when we don't want to see them again. Regressions to past behavior are common and tend to occur when your resilience, your ability to roll with the punches, is low due to lack of sleep, high levels of stress, sickness, and other challenges that exhaust your inner reserves (again recall the five S's from Chapter 5).

When a regression occurs, it is best to recognize it for what it is and not magnify it ("This is really a disaster—it's *awful!*") or catastrophize it ("Now things will be even worse than before!"). How you label or think about what has happened is what determines the impact of a regression on what you do next. Think of it as an expected reaction to stress and forgive yourself for being human. Most important, tell yourself you can get back on track by thinking through how you will react the next time your partner acts out his or her anger so you are again prepared for what is to come.

Setbacks Usually Begin in Your Head

The early warning alarm system for a setback is truly all in your head. Whether this setback is a result of not enough practice or the impact of stress-induced regression, the first thing you will be aware of are thoughts that seem to undermine your new behavior. Self-talk can either fuel a regression into becoming permanent (a true "back to base one") or inspire you to turn it around and stay the course. Your self-talk is very likely to precede your actions, and by staying alert and aware of how you're thinking, particularly when stressed, exhausted, or feeling that your partner's roadblocks are getting to you, you may be able to halt a setback in its tracks. Even if in your human fallibility you have "totally blown it" and returned to your old behavior for a day or more (a MAJOR setback), you can still get back on track by rethinking the situation rationally and reinstituting your original A–E strategy, fueled by this new thinking.

The table on the facing page shows examples of the self-talk experienced by the people described in this chapter, who all were eventually able to overcome obstacles thrown in their paths, even though most had setbacks. For each kind of unhelpful thought you will find a counter-thought you can adopt that promotes a confident and calm return to asserting boundaries. If you feel you are having a setback, look these over. Any sound familiar?

Unhelpful thoughts that fuel discomfort and a return to old behavior are a natural and common occurrence. To keep on top of a possible setback, continue your Daily Log to fuel personal awareness of how you are doing. Ask yourself these questions whenever it feels like things are slipping back to the way they were:

- **"Am I having thoughts that support my new boundaries or thoughts that seem to be undermining my efforts** [like those in the sidebar on page 70]? If so, I need to immediately write down the unhelpful thoughts so I can blow them away with rebuttals that focus on the **facts, how I need to feel**, and my **new plan."**

- **"Am I feeling confident and calmer as I am implementing my new boundaries, or am I returning to anxieties, anger, fear, or guilt?** If so, I need to immediately examine my thinking as above and take steps to reduce my stress: exercise, do something kind for myself (get a manicure, go to a movie, call or visit a close friend), practice a relaxation technique [like taking your deepest breath and then exhaling it as slowly as you can, tensing and then relaxing each muscle group]." Wonderful guides to help you manage stress are found in the Suggested Resources section at the back of the book.

- **"Are my new assertive behaviors starting to feel more automatic, or am I beginning to react as I once did?"** Stay aware of your old actions like editing, redirecting, placating, and rationalizing and immediately state to yourself what you need to do to stand up for your

Transforming Your Self-Talk

Setback-Inducing Self-Talk	Setback-Discouraging Self-Talk
"This is too overwhelming for me."	"I have handled a lot worse, like (when Dad died, I lost my job, etc.). I am strong and can do it!"
"I just can't change. I've been this way for too long."	"I have been changing my whole life as I took on new things (college, job, relationships) and can continue to change."
"I am harming our relationship by putting us through all this."	"I am changing how I react. My partner is putting us through this by his/her actions!"
"I've tried very hard, but this just isn't working."	"I cannot go back to the way things were. If I stay the course, things will change for me even if he/she does not change."
"He will never change, so why bother? It's hopeless!"	"I am powerless over what he decides to do, but I am hopeful that my changes will make my own life much better."
"When I feel stronger, I will try to do this, but not now."	"Strength and confidence come from acting, not waiting or trying. If I wait, I keep things as they are."
"I am too exhausted to get into an argument tonight. I'll start tomorrow."	"Getting rest is good, but I must not put off what I need to do."

new boundary. These self-instructions function as an inner guide that directs your next efforts. Do some rehearsals in your imagination to clearly define how you need to act the next time a challenging situation with your partner arises. Remember: the more you rehearse these new behaviors, the more they are grooved into your memory, like the ruts made by the wheels of a wagon on a dirt road.

While I have emphasized that obstacles and setbacks are to be expected along the new road you are traveling, please don't be intimidated. Standing up for your new boundaries is likely to have a profound impact on the quality of your life day to day and may well set the stage for your partner to get with it and embrace the kind of communication and intimacy you are hoping for. Regardless, you are on your way to new outcomes that better fit your vision of the kind of life you want to lead with your partner and for yourself.

Your self-esteem and sense of personal integrity are bound to grow as you no longer permit yourself to be treated with disrespect or contempt. You are setting your own course and inviting your partner to come along with you. Maybe he or she just will.

APPENDIX

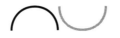

THE DAILY LOG

SITUATION (where, what did partner say or do?):

THOUGHTS (self-talk about your partner, yourself and why this happened?):

FEELINGS (anxious, guilty, angry, fearful?)

ACTIONS (what you did or said in response?):

OUTCOME (how did you end up feeling?, was the outcome positive or negative?):

YOUR PLAN IF THIS HAPPENS AGAIN?:

SUGGESTED RESOURCES

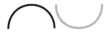

TO LEARN MORE ABOUT IDENTIFYING, UNDERSTANDING, AND MANAGING ANGER

Nay, W. R. (2004). *Taking charge of anger: How to resolve conflict, sustain relationships, and express yourself without losing control*. New York: Guilford Press.—Begins with a questionnaire to help you identify which face(s) of anger is a problem. In six steps the reader learns to recognize his or her specific anger profile, to recognize anger triggers, to reduce anger arousal, to challenge anger-fueling self-talk, and to communicate effectively without fueling conflict. A perfect companion to this book.

Nay, W. R. (2008). *The storm within—a workbook: Six steps to managing your anger*. Annapolis, MD: Self-published. Available at *www.wrobertnay.com*.

Harbin, T. J. (2000). *Beyond anger: A guide for men: How to free yourself from the grip of anger and get more out of life*. Philadelphia: Da Capo Press.

Tavris, C. (1989). *Anger: The misunderstood emotion*. New York: Touchstone Books.

Williams, R., & Williams, V. (1998). *Anger kills: Seventeen strategies for controlling the hostility that can harm your health*. New York: Harper.—An excellent review of how anger impacts your health by a leading researcher. Includes strategies to control hostility.

Website

W. Robert Nay
www.wrobertnay.com

Go to the "My Anger Advisor" section. To learn more about anger in your relationship, managing anger, or to seek personal coaching to guide your journey in addressing anger in your life or relationships, go to W. Robert Nay's website or contact him at wrnay@comcast.net.

FOR MORE INFORMATION ABOUT PASSIVE ANGER

Wetzler, S. (1993). *Living with the passive–aggressive man*. New York: Fireside Press.

Murphy, T., & Oberlin, L. H. (2005). *Overcoming passive–aggression: How to stop hidden anger from spoiling your relationships, career, and happiness*. New York: Wiley.

FOR MORE INFORMATION ABOUT VERBAL AND PHYSICAL ABUSE

Evans, P. (2003). *The verbally abusive relationship: How to recognize it and how to respond*. New York: Adams Media.

Evans, P. (2006). *The verbally abusive man, can he change?: A woman's guide to deciding whether to stay or go*. New York: Adams Media.

Engel, B. (2003). *The emotionally abusive relationship: How to stop being abused and how to stop abusing*. New York: Wiley.

Websites

Centers for Disease Control and Prevention
www.cdc.gov/injury

A rich compendium of information on intimate partner violence (IPV).

National Coalition against Domestic Violence (NCADV)
www.ncadv.org

Provides great information and a referral to local organizations that can offer help.

Halton Women's Place Safety Planning Checklist
www.haltonwomensplace.com/safety.htm

Rather than review the many books available on domestic violence, I refer you to this website, which continuously updates its listing of books on this topic. You can order online at a discount: *www.growing.com/accolade/viol/dfviol.htm*.

IF YOU FEEL YOU ARE IN DANGER

1. Call **911** and let the local police handle it.

2. Call the National Domestic Violence Hotline: **1-800-799-7233**.

IF DEPRESSION OR MOOD IS A FACTOR FOR YOU OR YOUR PARTNER

Burns, D. (1999). *Feeling good: The new mood therapy*. New York: Avon Books.—Many who have problems with anger also experience a mood disorder, which sometimes must be addressed with medication and therapy. This comprehensive book helps you assess whether you have a problem with depression and how to use cognitive-behavioral therapy to manage your mood. It also reviews the most common antidepressant medications.

Sheffield, A. (2003). *Depression fallout: The impact of depression on couples and what you can do to preserve the bond*. New York: Harper.—Very helpful in offering ideas on how to cope with your partner's depression (which may contribute to one or more faces of anger and make it hard to communicate).

Strauss, C. J. (2004). *Talking to depression: Simple ways to connect when someone in your life is depressed*. New York: NAL Trade.

Websites

For information on the role of anger in health or any other question related to mental health, go to:

Mental Health Net-Self-Help Resources
mentalhelp.net/selfhelp.htm

Depression support
www.onelist.com/community/rosesandthorns or *www.onelist.com/community/melancholy*
    If you or someone you care about is experiencing a mood disorder that affects anger and relationships, either of these websites is excellent.

Psych Central
psychcentral.com

IF STRESS IS A FACTOR FOR YOU OR YOUR PARTNER

It is imperative to manage daily anxiety and stress that lowers your resilience, making you vulnerable when the next difficult situation comes along. These resources can help you set some new goals for managing your day.

Charlesworth, E., & Nathan, R. G. (2004). *Stress management: A comprehensive guide to wellness.* New York: Ballantine Books.

Bourne, E. (2005). *The anxiety and phobia workbook* (4th ed.). Oakland, CA: New Harbinger.—An outstanding treatment manual offering numerous ideas for managing all forms of anxiety—all of which can make you more susceptible to an anger episode.

Davis, M., Eschelman, E., McKay, M., & Fanning, P. (2008). *The relaxation and stress reduction workbook.* Oakland, CA: New Harbinger.—An award-winning presentation of all the common techniques used for relaxation and stress management. Written in clear language and easy to read. Highly recommended.

Website

American Institute of Stress

www.stress.org

Provides comprehensive information and resources for identifying and managing stress at home and at work.

IF LACK OF SLEEP SEEMS TO MAKE THINGS WORSE

Sleep deprivation often fuels irritability and lowers mood. If you or your partner find it difficult to get required levels of sleep, these books may help you assess whether you have a sleep problem that can be helped by medical treatment. Regardless, numerous well-researched ideas for changing your sleep schedule are offered.

Epstein, L., & Marden, S. (2006). *The Harvard Medical School guide to a good night's sleep.* New York: McGraw-Hill.

Dement, W. C. (2000). *The promise of sleep: A pioneer in sleep medicine explores the vital connection between health, happiness, and a good night's sleep.* New York: Dell Books.—A well-regarded sleep researcher describes the kinds of sleep problems you may be experiencing, teaches you to assess your own sleep habits, and then offers a "sleep-smart" lifestyle and tips for getting a good night's sleep.

If your child's sleep problems are affecting your own night's sleep, this book offers ideas from pediatricians for getting your child to settle down and sleep.

Cohen, G. J. (Ed.). (2002). *American Academy of Pediatrics guide to your child's sleep.* New York: Villard Books.

Websites

Both of these websites provide an extraordinary amount of information about fostering good sleep and assessing and treating sleep disorders.

Sleepnet
www.sleepnet.com

American Academy of Sleep Medicine
www.aasmnet.org
    This site offers sleep information for both professional and public consumers.

IF ALCOHOL OR SUBSTANCE ABUSE SEEMS TO FUEL CONFLICT

Overuse or addiction to alcohol or substances greatly increases the likelihood of losing control of your anger. Each of these references may be helpful to your partner or you in assessing and altering the use of substances or give you ideas to encourage someone you care about to seek help.

Cornett, D. J. (2005). *Seven weeks to safe social drinking: How to effectively moderate your alcohol intake.* New York: People Friendly Books.—If your partner objects to abstaining completely from alcohol, this program will help him or her reduce alcohol intake that can fuel anger intensity. If your partner cannot effectively moderate drinking, then abstinence and a wonderful program like Alcoholics Anonymous is the answer.

Ketcham, K., & Asbury, W. F. (2000). *Beyond the influence: Understanding and defeating alcoholism.* New York: Bantam Doubleday.—Updating the seminal book *Under the Influence*, chapters review the impact of alcohol use on health, stages of an alcohol problem, and ideas for sustaining abstinence. A good book to read if you wonder if you have a problem.

Santoro, J., Bergman, A., & Deletis, R. (2001). *Kill the craving: How to control the impulse to use drugs and alcohol.* Oakland, CA: New Harbinger.—Details specific strategies for using exposure and response therapy to manage urges to use substances. Clearly written workbook format.

Websites

Join Together
www.jointogether.org
 A thorough listing of alcohol and substance abuse information.

PrevLine: National Clearinghouse for Alcohol and Drug Information
www.health.org
 A wealth of fact sheets, the latest in research, and many online resources are provided, along with a great search engine to satisfy your specific questions.

TO LEARN MORE
ABOUT IMPROVING COMMUNICATION

Gottman, J. (1995). *Why marriages succeed and fail: And how you can make yours last.* New York: Simon & Schuster.

McKay, M., & Fanning, P. (2006). *Couples skills: Making your relationship work.* San Francisco: New Harbinger.

Tannen, D. (2001). *You just don't understand: Women and men in conversation.* New York: Quill.—A noted linguist reviews research on how men and women communicate very differently and how to improve effective communication with your partner.

Stone, D., Patton, B., Heen, S., & Fisher, R. (2000). *Difficult conversations: How to discuss what matters most.* New York: Penguin Books.—Based on the Harvard Negotiation Project, the authors help you prepare yourself for communicating with difficult people on difficult subjects, while defusing conflict and achieving resolution.

Websites

Couples' Communication Program
www.couplecommunication.com
 Since 1972 Dr. Sherrod Miller and colleagues have offered a wonderful program, first developed at the University of Minnesota, to reduce conflict and improve communication in relationships.

Smart Marriages
www.smartmarriages.com
 This organization holds a well-attended conference each year to present the latest in treatment and assessment of marriages. Its website offers articles, recommended programs, and the latest research for the lay public.

ASSOCIATIONS AND ORGANIZATIONS
YOU MIGHT FIND USEFUL

In addition to the organizations and websites already mentioned, each of these provides useful information, readings, treatment recommendations, and other valuable data. Each has a search engine for locating specific topics (e.g., anger management, stress disorders). Websites to get you quickly to the public information they offer are listed for each.

American Association of Marriage and Family Therapy
112 South Alfred Street
Alexandria, VA 22314-3061
www.aamft.org

American Psychiatric Association—Public Information
1000 Wilson Boulevard, Suite 1825
Arlington, VA 22209-3901
www.psych.org/public_info

American Psychological Association
750 First Street, NE
Washington, DC 20002-4242
www.apa.org

American Psychological Association Help Center
www.helping.apa.org

Coalition for Marriage, Family and Couples
5310 Belt Road, NW
Washington, DC 20015-1961
www.smartmarriages.com

National Alliance on Mental Illness
Colonial Place Three
2107 Wilson Boulevard, Suite 300
Arlington, VA 22201
www.nami.org

National Institute of Mental Health
6001 Executive Boulevard, Room 8184
Bethesda, MD 20892-9663
www.nimh.nih.gov/health/publications

National Mental Health Association
2001 North Beauregard Street, 12th Floor
Alexandria, VA 22311
www.nmha.org

BIBLIOGRAPHY

Alberti, R. E., & Emmons, M. L. (2001). *Your perfect right: Assertiveness and equality in your life and relationships* (8th ed.). New York: Impact.

American Psychological Association. (1996). *Violence and the family.* Washington, DC: Author.

Branson, R. (1988). *Coping with difficult people.* New York: Anchor Press/Doubleday.

Burns, D. (1999). *Feeling good: The new mood therapy.* New York: Avon Books.

Caetano, R., Schafer, J., & Cunradi, C. B. (2001). Alcohol-related intimate partner violence among white, black, and Hispanic couples in the United States. *Alcohol Research and Health, 25,* 58–65.

Cassidy, J., & Shaver, P. R. (Eds.). (2009). *Handbook of attachment* (2nd ed.). New York: Guilford Press.

Centers for Disease Control and Prevention. (2008). *Intimate partner violence: Consequences.* Atlanta, GA: CDC National Center for Injury Prevention.

Dutton, D. G. (2008). *The abusive personality: Violence and control in intimate relationships* (2nd ed.). New York: Guilford Press.

Feindler, E. L., Rathus, J., & Silver, B. (2003). *Assessment of family violence.* Washington, DC: American Psychological Association.

Geffner, R., & Rosenbaum, A. (1990). Characteristics and treatment of batterers. *Behavioral Sciences and the Law, 8,* 131–140.

Gottman, J. M. (1985). *Why marriages succeed and fail.* New York: Fireside Books.

Gottman, J. M. (1999). *The marriage clinic.* New York: Norton.

Holloway, J. D. (2003). Advances in anger management. *APA Monitor, 34*(3), 54.

Jacobson, N. S., & Gottman, J. M. (1998). *When men batter women.* New York: Simon & Schuster.

Kassinove, H., & Tafrate, C. (2002). *Anger management: The complete treatment guidebook for practitioners*. New York: Impact Press.

Kaufman Kantor, G., & Asdigian, N. (1997). Gender differences in alcohol-related spousal aggression. In R. Wilsnack & S. Wilsnack (Eds.), *Gender and alcohol: Individual and social perspectives* (pp. 312–334). New Brunswick, NJ: Rutgers Center of Alcohol Studies.

Lawson, D. M. (2003). Incidence, explanations, and treatment of partner violence. *Journal of Counseling and Development, 81*, 19–52.

Lerner, H. G. (1985). *The dance of anger*. New York: Harper & Row.

Margolin, G., John, R. S., & Foo, L. (1998). Interactive and unique risk factors for husbands' emotional and physical abuse of their wives. *Journal of Family Violence, 13*, 315–345.

Meichenbaum, D. (1985). *Stress inoculation training*. New York: Allyn & Bacon.

Murphy, T., & Oberlin, L. H. (2005). *Overcoming passive–aggression: How to stop hidden anger from spoiling your relationships, career and happiness*. Philadelphia: Da Capo Press.

National Coalition Against Domestic Violence. (2009). *Domestic violence facts*. Washington, DC: NCADV Public Policy Office.

National Women's Health Information Center. (2008). *Safety planning list*. Washington, DC: U.S. Department of Health and Human Services.

Nay, W. R. (1995). Anger and aggression: Cognitive-behavioral and short-term interventions. In L. Vandercreek, S. Knap, & T. Jackson (Eds.), *Innovations in clinical practice* (pp. 111–136). Sarasota, FL: Professional Resources Press.

Nay, W. R. (2004). *Taking charge of anger: How to resolve conflict, sustain relationships, and express yourself without losing control*. New York: Guilford Press.

Neidig, P. H., & Friedman, D. H. (1984). *Spouse abuse: A treatment program for couples*. Champaign, IL: Research Press.

O'Leary, K. D., Barling, J., Arias, I., Rosenbaum, A., Malone, J., & Tyree, A. (1989). Prevalence and stability of physical aggression between spouses: A longitudinal analysis. *Journal of Consulting and Clinical Psychology, 57*, 263–268.

O'Leary, K. D., & Woodin, E. M. (2009). *Psychological and physical aggression in couples: Causes and interventions*. Washington, DC: American Psychological Association.

Patterson, G. R. (1982). *Coercive family process*. Eugene, OR: Castalia.

Pollack, W. (1999). *Real boys*. New York: Owl Books.

Rosenman, R. H., & Friedman, M. (1971). The possible role of behavior patterns in proneness and immunity to coronary heart disease. In H. I. Russek & B. L. Zolman (Eds.), *Coronary heart disease* (pp. 210–221). Philadelphia: Lippincott.

Rugala, E. A., & Isaacs, A. R. (2004). *Workplace violence: Issues in response*. Quantico, VA: National Center for the Analysis of Violent Crime, FBI Academy.

Tannen, D. (1990). *You just don't understand: Women and men in conversation*. New York: Ballantine Books.

Tannen, D. (1999). *The argument culture: Stopping America's war of words.* New York: Ballantine Books.

Tavris, C. (1989). *Anger: The misunderstood emotion.* New York: Touchstone Books.

Weisz, A. N., Tolman, R. M., & Saunders, D. G. (2000). Assessing the risk of severe domestic violence: The importance of survivors' predictions. *Journal of Interpersonal Violence, 15,* 75–90.

Wetzler, S. (1993). *Living with the passive–aggressive man.* New York: Fireside Books.

Whitaker, D. J., & Lutzker, J. R. (2009). *Preventing partner violence: Research and evidence-based intervention strategies.* Washington, DC: American Psychological Association.

Williams, R., & Williams, V. (1998). *Anger kills: Seventeen strategies for controlling the hostility that can harm your health.* New York: Harper.

INDEX

Hypervigilance
  anxiety and, 31
  hostility and, 115
  overview, 115

I
"I" message. *See also* Communication
  active listening and, 99–100, 101
  defusing provocation and, 100,
    102–103
  hostility and, 125
  overview, 22, 97–103
  passive anger and, 193, 194, 202–203,
    205
  violence and, 170, 175–176, 177
Illness
  anger arousal and, 97
  resistance from your partner and,
    215–216
Impact of anger, 12–17
Incompetence excuse roadblock,
  218–219
Indirect anger. *See* Passive anger
Inner comments, 74. *See also* Self-talk
Instrumental aggression, 157–159. *See
  also* Aggression
Insults, 137–140. *See also* Contempt;
  Verbal aggression
Interrupting behavior, 44
Intimacy, withholding. *See also* Passive
    anger; Withdrawal
  affirmation needs and, 51
  needs and, 56
  overview, 185
  passive anger and, 187
Intimidation, 161–162

J
Journalling. *See* Daily log
Justifying anger in others. *See also*
    Excuses for anger
  angry response to anger and, 37–38
  denial of rewards step and, 90–91
  hostility and, 120
  overview, 2–3, 90–91
  problems with, 9–10
  Relationship Anger Profile (RAP)
    questionnaire and, 29–30

K
Kicking. *See* Aggression; Violence

L
Lateness, 187–188
Leaving, needs and, 56
Legitimacy, as an excuse or
    rationalization, 35
Limit setting, 21–22. *See also* Boundaries

Listening skills
  active listening, 99–100, 101, 218–219
  expressing yourself effectively step
    and, 92–93
  resistance from your partner and,
    218–219
Log, daily. *See* Daily log
Loudness, 44

M
Medical issues
  hostility and, 127–128
  resistance from your partner and,
    215–216
Medicalizing roadblock, 215–216
Mental disorders, 167
Minimizing
  examples of, 171
  hostility and, 122
  overview, 75–76
  resistance from your partner and,
    220, 226
  violence and, 171
Mirroring, 100
Mood factors, 239. *See also* Depression
Musculoskeletal responses, 32

N
Name-calling. *See also* Verbal aggression
  boundaries and, 144–147
  development of violence and, 166
  overview, 132–133
Narcissism
  aggression and, 158
  hostility and, 128
  violence and, 167
National Coalition against Domestic
    Violence (NCADV), 145
Needs. *See also* Achievement need;
    Affirmation; Control needs; Safety;
    Security
  boundaries and, 49–61
  getting your needs met and, 54–61
  "I" message and, 98–99
  resistance from your partner and, 227
Negative labeling. *See also* Verbal
    aggression
  boundaries and, 144–147
  overview, 140–141

O
Outbursts, 56
Overgeneralizing roadblock, 214–215

P
Pain
  hostility and, 127–128
  resistance from your partner and,
    215–216

ABOUT THE AUTHOR

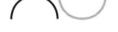

W. Robert Nay, PhD, is a clinical psychologist in private practice in McLean, Virginia, and Annapolis, Maryland, and Clinical Associate Professor at Georgetown University School of Medicine. He has trained thousands of mental health professionals nationwide to work on anger management and relationship issues with their clients. The author of *Taking Charge of Anger,* Dr. Nay lives in Annapolis with his wife. His website is *www.wrobertnay.com.*